Taste Masked Oral Distinguishing Tablets of Tolterodine Tartrate

Shravan Kumar Yamsani
Sathish Dharani
Jairaj Pothula

Taste Masked Oral Distinguishing Tablets of Tolterodine Tartrate

Scholar's Press

Impressum / Imprint

Bibliografische Information der Deutschen Nationalbibliothek: Die Deutsche Nationalbibliothek verzeichnet diese Publikation in der Deutschen Nationalbibliografie; detaillierte bibliografische Daten sind im Internet über http://dnb.d-nb.de abrufbar.

Alle in diesem Buch genannten Marken und Produktnamen unterliegen warenzeichen-, marken- oder patentrechtlichem Schutz bzw. sind Warenzeichen oder eingetragene Warenzeichen der jeweiligen Inhaber. Die Wiedergabe von Marken, Produktnamen, Gebrauchsnamen, Handelsnamen, Warenbezeichnungen u.s.w. in diesem Werk berechtigt auch ohne besondere Kennzeichnung nicht zu der Annahme, dass solche Namen im Sinne der Warenzeichen- und Markenschutzgesetzgebung als frei zu betrachten wären und daher von jedermann benutzt werden dürften.

Bibliographic information published by the Deutsche Nationalbibliothek: The Deutsche Nationalbibliothek lists this publication in the Deutsche Nationalbibliografie; detailed bibliographic data are available in the Internet at http://dnb.d-nb.de.

Any brand names and product names mentioned in this book are subject to trademark, brand or patent protection and are trademarks or registered trademarks of their respective holders. The use of brand names, product names, common names, trade names, product descriptions etc. even without a particular marking in this works is in no way to be construed to mean that such names may be regarded as unrestricted in respect of trademark and brand protection legislation and could thus be used by anyone.

Coverbild / Cover image: www.ingimage.com

Verlag / Publisher:
Scholar's Press
ist ein Imprint der / is a trademark of
AV Akademikerverlag GmbH & Co. KG
Heinrich-Böcking-Str. 6-8, 66121 Saarbrücken, Deutschland / Germany
Email: info@scholars-press.com

Herstellung: siehe letzte Seite /
Printed at: see last page
ISBN: 978-3-639-51440-7

Zugl. / Approved by: Vaagdevi College of Pharmacy, Kakatiya University

Copyright © 2013 AV Akademikerverlag GmbH & Co. KG
Alle Rechte vorbehalten. / All rights reserved. Saarbrücken 2013

TABLE OF CONTENTS

No. of Chapter	Page No.
1. INTRODUCTION	3
1.1. Oral disintegrating tablets (ODTs)	3
1.2. Various technologies used in the manufacture of ODTs	7
1.3. Patented technologies for oral disintegrating tablets	15
1.4. Role of super disintegrants in ODTs	22
1.5. Mechanism of Super disintegrants	23
2. METHODOLOGY	30
2.1. Preparation of standard graph of Tolterodine Tartrate in 0.1NHCl	30
2.2. Preparation of standard graph of Tolterodine Tartrate in pH 6.8 Phoshpate buffer	30
2.3. Preparation of Drug - Polymer Complex	30
2.4. Preparation of Tolterodine Tartrate ODTs by direct compression technique	31
2.5. Evaluation of DPC drug content and *in-Vitro* taste evaluation	33
2.6. Evaluation of orally disintegration tablet formulations	33
3. **RESULTS**	37
4. **DISCUSSION**	59
5. **CONCLUSIONS**	63
REFERENCES	

PURPOSE OF STUDY

Oral administration is the most popular route while compared to other dosage forms due to ease of ingestion, pain avoidance, versatility and most importantly patient compliance. One important drawback of solid dosage forms is the difficulty in swallowing (dysphasia) or chewing in some patients particularly pediatric and geriatric patients.

Therefore, ODTs would serves as an ideal dosage form for patients with difficulty in swallowing of tablets and hard gelatin capsules. These dosage forms are designed in such a way that they disintegrate or dissolve in patient's mouth upon contact with saliva, within seconds without aid of water. Drug then enters the stomach as finer particles which may get rapidly dissolved in the gastric fluid due to the larger surface area of the drug particles which increases absorption leading to faster onset of action.

PLAN OF WORK

The aim of the present study is to develop taste masked orally disintegrating tablets of Tolterodine Tartrate to achieve rapid disintegration ant to provide rapid onset of action. Also to resolve the swallowing problems in pediatric, geriatric patients by rapid disintegration in saliva and improve the patient compliance. The Tolterodine Tartrate orally disintegrating tablets are prepared by using different super disintegrants like crosspovidone, croscarmellose sodium, sodium starch glycolate, at different concentrations and diluents microcrystalline cellulose pH 102. The effect of superdisintegrants were evaluated by *in vitro* and *in vivo* disintegration time and also on the *in vitro* drug release was observed.

STUDY PROTOCOL

1. To prepare oral disintegrating tablets by direct compression method.

2. Construction of standard graph of Tolterodine Tartrate in 0.1NHCl.

3. Preparation of Drug-Polymer complex (DPC).

4. Determination of Drug content in Drug-Polymer complex.

5. In Vitro taste evaluation of Drug-Polymer complex.

6. Preparation of Orodispersible Tablets using different concentrations of superdisintegrants.

7. Characterization of Drug-Polymer complex by Fourier transform infrared spectroscopy.

8. The oral disintegrating tablets are to be characterized for the following parameters:
   a. Weight variation
   b. Thickness
   c. Hardness
   d. Friability
   e. Drug content
   f. Wetting time
   g. Water absorption ratio
   h. *In vitro* Disintegration time
   i. *In vivo* Disintegration time
   j. Taste evaluation
   k. Dissolution study

1. INTRODUCTION

1.1. Oral disintegrating tablets (ODTs)

Among the available pharmaceutical dosage forms, tablets are the most widely used dosage form because of their convenience in terms of self medication, ease of administration, accurate dosage, compactness, good stability and ease of manufacturing. The Elderly constitute a major portion of world population today. These people will experience deterioration of their physiological and physical abilities like dysphagia (difficulty in swallowing). Pediatric patients may suffer from ingestion problems of their underdeveloped muscular and nervous system (Shery et al., 2009). In order to overcome this problem, a new drug delivery system has been developed known as Orally Disintegrating Tablets (ODTs). Orally Disintegrating Tablets are solid dosage form containing medicinal substances which disintegrates/dissolves rapidly upon contact with saliva. When these tablets are placed in oral cavity, saliva penetrates into the pores causing rapid disintegration. These tablets are beneficial for the patients suffering from nausea and vomiting, those with mental disorders, bedridden and those who do not have easy access of water.

US Food and Drug Administration Center for Drug Evaluation and Research (CDER) defines, in the 'Orange Book', an ODT as "A solid dosage form containing medicinal substances, which disintegrates rapidly, usually within a matter of seconds, when placed upon the tongue".

Recently European Pharmacopoeia used the term 'Orodispersible tablet' as a tablet that is to be placed in the mouth where it disperses rapidly before swallowing.

Orally disintegrating tablets are also called as mouth-dissolving tablets, fast disintegrating tablets, fast dissolving tablets, orodispersible tablets, rapimelts, porous tablets, quick dissolving tablet (Madhusudan Rao et al., 2008).

The US Food and Drug Administration responded to this challenge with the 2008 publication of Guidance for Industry Orally Disintegrating Tablets (Rosie et al., 2009). Three main points stand out in the final guidance:

- ODTs should have an *in vitro* disintegration time of approximately 30 s or less.
- Generally, the ODT tablet weight should not exceed 500 mg, although the combined influence of tablet weight, size and component solubility all factor into the acceptability of an ODT for both patients and regulators.

- The guidance serves to define the upper limits of the ODT category, but it does not supersede or replace the original regulatory definition mentioned. In other words, disintegration within a matter of seconds remains the target for an ODT.

1.1.1. Advantages of Orally disintegrating tablets:
- ODTs includes both the advantages of solid and liquid formulations such as good stability, accurate dosing, easy manufacturing, small packaging size, and easy handling by patients and no risk of suffocation resulting from physical obstruction by a dosage form (Tejvir et al., 2011).
- Increased bioavailability, because the tablets disintegrate inside the mouth, drugs may be absorbed in the buccal pharyngeal and gastric region which results in pre-gastric absorption, thereby avoiding first-pass metabolism.
- API side effects may be avoided if they are caused by first-pass effect.
- The advantage of ODTs is administration without water under circumstances like travelling and working.
- Rapid disintegration of the tablet results in quick dissolution and rapid absorption thereby providing provide rapid onset of action.
- The risk of chocking or suffocation during oral administration of conventional formulation due to physical obstruction is avoided, thus providing improved safety (Debjit et al., 2009).
- Good mouth feel property of ODTs helps to change the perception of medication as bitter pill particularly in pediatric patient.
- Beneficial in cases such as motion sickness, sudden episodes of allergic attack or coughing, where an ultra rapid onset of action required.
- New business opportunities: product differentiation, line extension and life-cycle management, exclusivity of product promotion and patent-life extension.

1.1.2. Limitations of ODTs:
- The tablets usually have insufficient mechanical strength. Hence, careful handling is required.
- The tablets may leave unpleasant taste and grittiness in mouth if not formulated properly (Rakesh et al., 2010).

1.1.3. Challenges to develop ODTs:
- Rapid disintegration of tablet

- Avoid increase in tablet size
- Have sufficient mechanical strength
- Minimum or no residue in mouth
- Protection from moisture
- Good package design
- Compatible with taste masking technology
- Not affected by drug properties (Suresh et al., 2008).

1.1.4. Selection of drug candidates for ODTs:

Several factors must be considered while selecting drug candidates for delivery as ODT dosage forms (William et al., 2005). The ultimate characteristics of a drug for dissolution in the mouth and pre gastric absorption from ODTs include

- Free from bitter taste.
- Dose should be low as possible.
- Small to moderate molecular weight.
- Good solubility in water and saliva.
- Partially non – ionized at oral cavity's pH.
- Patients who concurrently take anti-cholinergic medications may not be the best candidates for these drugs.
- ODTs formulations cannot be used in Patients with Sjogren's syndrome or dryness of the mouth due to decreased saliva production.
- Drugs with a short half-life and frequent dosing may not be suitable for ODTs.
- Drugs which are having very bitter taste may not be suitable for ODTs taste masking cannot be achieved.
- Drugs which require controlled or sustained release are unsuitable candidates of fast dissolving oral dosage forms.

1.1.5. Selection of Superdisintegrants:

Superdisintegrants not only affect the rate of disintegration, but when used at higher concentrations they can also affect mouth feel, tablet hardness and friability (Rakes et al., 2010). Hence, various ideal factors to be considered while selecting appropriate superdisintegrants for a particular formulation should.

- Produce rapid disintegration.
- Be compactable enough to produce less-friable tablets.
- Produce good mouth feel to the patient. Thus, small particle size is preferred to achieve patient compliance.
- Should have good flow properties to improve the flow ability of the total blend.

Some of the superdisintegrants are:

1. **Sodium Starch Glycolate (Explotab, primogel):** It is used in concentration of 2-8 % & optimum is 4%.

   Mechanism of Action: Rapid and extensive swelling with minimal gelling and water wicking.

2. **Cross-linked Povidone (crospovidone)** used in concentration of 2-5% of weight of tablet completely insoluble in water.

   Mechanism of Action: Water wicking, swelling and possibly some deformation recovery. Rapidly disperses and swells in water, but does not gel even after prolonged exposure. Greatest rate of swelling compared to other disintegrants Greater surface area to volume ratio than other disintegrants.

3. **Cross linked carboxymethylcellulose sodium (Croscarmellose sodium)**

   Mechanism of Action: Wicking due to fibrous structure, swelling with minimal gelling effective concentrations 1-3% direct compression, 2-4% Wet granulation.

1.1.6. Ideal properties of Orally disintegrating tablets:

- Orally disintegrating tablets should not require water to swallow and should dissolve or disintegrate in the mouth within a few seconds (Rakesh et al., 2010).
- Allow high drug loading.
- Be compatible with taste masking and other excipients.
- Have a pleasing mouth feel.
- Leave minimal or no residue in the mouth after oral administration.
- Have sufficient strength to withstand the rigors of the manufacturing process and post manufacturing handling.
- Exhibit low sensitivity to environmental conditions such as humidity and temperature.
- Be adaptable and amenable to existing processing and packaging machinery.

- Allow the manufacture of tablets using conventional processing and packaging equipments at low cost.

1.1.7. Formulation aspects in developing ODTs:

Orally disintegrating tablets are formulated by utilizing several processes, which differ in their methodologies and ODTs formed vary in various properties such as (Suresh et al., 2008).

1. Mechanical strength of tablets
2. Taste and mouth feel
3. Swallow ability
4. Drug dissolution in saliva
5. Bioavailability
6. Stability

1.2. Various technologies used in the manufacture of odts:

The performance of ODT depends on the technology used in their manufacture. The orally disintegrating property of the tablet is attributable to a quick ingress of water into the tablet matrix, which creates porous structure and results in rapid disintegration. Hence, the basic approaches to develop ODT include maximizing the porous structure of the tablet matrix, incorporating the appropriate disintegrating agent & using highly water-soluble excipients in the formulation (Shukla et al., 2008). Following technologies have been used by various researchers to prepare ODTs:

1. Freeze drying or Lyophilization
2. Spray drying
3. Molding
4. Phase transition process
5. Melt granulation
6. Sublimation
7. Mass extrusion
8. Cotton candy process
9. Direct compression
10. Nanonization
11. Effervescent method

1.2.1. Freeze-Drying or Lyophilization:

Freeze drying (lyophilization) is a process in which solvent is removed from a frozen drug solution or a suspension containing structure-forming excipients. The resulting tablets are usually very light and have highly porous structures that allow rapid dissolution or disintegration. When placed on the tongue, the freeze dried unit dissolves almost instantly to release the incorporated drug. The entire freeze drying process is done at non elevated temperatures to eliminate adverse thermal effects that may affect drug stability during processing.

The tablets prepared by lyophilization disintegrate rapidly in less than 5 sec due to quick penetration of saliva in pores when placed in the oral cavity. Lyophilization is useful for heat sensitive drugs i.e. thermo-labile substances (Manoj et al., 2010).

A typical procedure involved in the manufacturing of ODT using this technique is mentioned here. The active drug is dissolved or dispersed in an aqueous solution of a carrier/polymer. The mixture is dosed by weight and poured in the wells of the preformed blister packs. The trays holding the blister packs are passed through liquid nitrogen freezing tunnel to freeze the drug solution or dispersion. Then the frozen blister packs are placed in refrigerated cabinets to continue the freeze-drying. After freeze-drying the aluminum foil backing is applied on a blister-sealing machine. Finally the blisters are packaged and shipped.

The freeze-drying technique has demonstrated improved absorption and increase in bioavailability. The major disadvantages of lyophillization technique are that it is expensive and time consuming fragility makes conventional packaging unsuitable for these products and poor stability under stressed conditions (Guptha et al., 2010).

1.2.2. Spray drying:

Spray drying methods are widely used in pharmaceutical and biochemical processes. Spray drying provides a fast and economical way of removing solvents and producing highly porous, fine powders. Spray drying can be used to prepare rapidly disintegrating tablets. This technique is based on a particulate support matrix, which is prepared by spray drying an aqueous composition containing support matrix and other components to form a highly porous and fine powder. This is then mixed with active ingredients and compressed into tablet (Kuldeep et al., 2010). Allen et al used a spray drying technique to prepare fast dissolving tablets. The tablets made from this technology are claimed to disintegrate within 20 seconds.

1.2.3. Molding:

Molded tablets disintegrate more rapidly and offer improved taste due to water soluble sugars present in dispersion matrix. Different molding techniques can be used to prepare orally disintegrating tablets

a. Compression molding (solvent method): The manufacturing process of molding tablets involves moistening the powder blend with a solvent (usually ethanol or water), and then the mixture is molded into tablets under pressures lower than those used in conventional tablet compression (Yourong et al., 2004). The solvent is then removed by air drying. Because molded tablets are usually compressed at a lower pressure than conventional compressed tablets, a higher porous structure is created to enhance the dissolution.

b. Heat molding: A molten matrix in which drug is dissolved or dispersed can be directly molded into orally disintegrating tablets. The tablets prepared using heat molding process involves settling of molten mass that contains a dispersed or dissolved drug (Manoj et al., 2010). The heat-molding process uses an agar solution as a binder and a blister packaging well as a mold to manufacture a tablet. The process involves preparing a suspension that contains a drug, agar, and sugar (e.g., Mannitol or lactose), pouring the suspension into the blister packaging well, solidifying the agar solution at room temperature to form a jelly, and drying at -30°C under vacuum (Tejvir et al., 2011).

C. No-vacuum lyophilization: The process involves the evaporation of solvent from a drug solution or suspension at standard pressure. Pebley et al., evaporated a frozen mixture containing a gum (e.g., acacia, carageenan, guar, tragacanth, or xanthan), a carbohydrate (e.g., dextrose, lactose, maltose, mannitol, or maltodextrin), and a solvent in a tablet shaped mould. Molded tablets typically do not possess great mechanical strength. Erosion and breakage of the molded tablet often occur during handling and opening of blister packs. In order to overcome this problem, binding agent such as sucrose, acacia, or polyvinyl pyrrolidone must be added to the solvent system, but then the rate of tablet solubility usually decreases. ODTs, having both adequate mechanical strength and good disintegration, recently have been prepared by molding techniques using nonconventional equipment and/ or multistep processes. The nonconventional approach, however, does cost more. Compared with freeze drying, ODTs prepared by molding techniques can be produced more simply and efficiently at an industrial scale, although they cannot achieve disintegration times comparable with those of lyophilized forms (Manoj et al., 2010).

1.2.4. Phase transition process:

The combination of low and high melting point sugar alcohols, as well as a phase transition in the manufacturing process, is important for making orally disintegrating tablets without any special apparatus. Here, tablets produced by compressing the powder containing two sugar alcohols of high and low melting point and subsequently heating at temperature between their two melting points. ODT's were produced by compressing powder containing erythritol (melting point: 122^0C) and xylitol (melting point 93 - 95^0C) and then heating at about 93^0C for 15min. After heating the median pore size of the tablets was increased and tablet hardness was also increased. The increase of tablet hardness with heating and storage did not depend on the crystal state of the lower melting point of the sugar alcohol (Manoj et al., 2010). Before heating process, tablet did not have sufficient hardness because of low compatibility but after heating, increase in inter particular bonding or binding surface area occurs which then increased tablet hardness.

1.2.5. Melt granulation:

Melt granulation technique is a process by which pharmaceutical powders are efficiently agglomerated by a meltable binder. The advantage of this technique compared to a conventional granulation is that no water or organic solvents is needed. Because there is no drying step, the process is less time consuming and uses less energy than wet granulation. It is a useful technique to enhance the dissolution rate of poorly water-soluble drugs, such as griseofulvin.

Oral disintegrating tablets was prepared by incorporating a hydrophilic waxy binder (super polystate) PEG- 6-Sterate. Superpolystate is a waxy material with a melting point of $33-37^0C$ and hydrophilic lipophilic balance of 9. It is not only acts as a binder and increases the physical resistance of tablets, but also helps the disintegration of tablets as it melts in the mouth and solubilizes rapidly leaving no residue in oral cavity (Abdelbary et al., 2009).
.Carbamazepine fast release tablets were prepared by melt granulation technique using PEG – 4000 as a melting binder and lactose monohydrate as hydrophilic filler.

1.2.6. Sublimation:

Sublimation has been used to produce ODTs with high porosity. A porous matrix is formed by compressing the volatile ingredients along with other excipients into tablets, which are finally subjected to a process of sublimation. Removal of volatile material by sublimation creates pores in tablet structure, due to which tablet dissolves when comes in contact with saliva. Inert solid ingredients with high volatility (e.g., ammonium bicarbonate, ammonium carbonate, benzoic acid, camphor, hexamethylene tetramine, naphthalene, phthalic anhydride, urea and urethene) have been used for this purpose (Rangasamy et al., 2009). Solvents such as cyclohexane and benzene were also suggested for generating the porosity in the matrix. Mouth dissolving tablets with highly porous structure and good mechanical strength have been developed by this method. These compressed tablets which have high porosity (approximately 30%) rapidly dissolved within 15 seconds in saliva.

Oral disintegrating tablets were developed by utilizing camphor a subliming material that is removed from compressed tablets prepared using a mixture of mannitol and camphor. Camphor was sublimated in vaccum at 80°C for 30 min after preparation of tablets.

Fast-dissolving tablet were developed by using water as the pore-forming material. A mixture containing an active ingredient and a carbohydrate (preferably sucrose, glucose, xylitol, or erythritol) was moistened with water (1-3% by weight) and compressed into tablets. The water was then removed, yielding highly porous tablets that exhibited excellent mechanical strength and a high dissolution rate (Kuldeep et al., 2010).

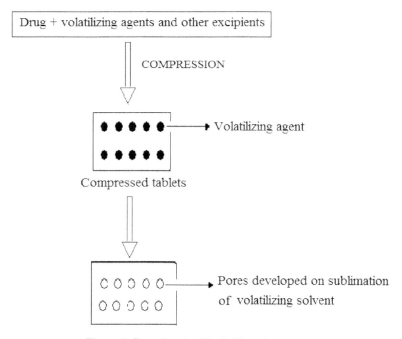

Figure 1. Steps Involved in Sublimation

1.2.7. Mass-Extrusion:

This technology involves softening the active blend using the solvent mixture of water soluble polyethylene glycol and methanol and expulsion of softened mass through the extruder or syringe to get a cylinder of the product into even segments using heated blade to form tablet. The dried cylinder can also be used to coat granules for bitter drugs and thereby achieve taste masking (Debjith et al., 2009).

1.2.8. Cotton candy process:

The cotton candy process is also known as the "candy floss" process and forms the basis of the technologies such as Flash Dose (Fuisz Technology). There are various pre blend mixtures used in the manufacture of 'floss', few of which are summarized in table1.1.

Table 1. Various preblend compositions used in floss process

Floss pre blend compositions	Drugs
Sucrose (78.25%), Sorbitol (11%), Xylitol (10%) and Tween 80 (0.75%)	Ibuprofen, Cimitedine, Vitamine C, Calcium carbonate/Vitamine D or Acetaminophen
Sucrose (84.5%), Mannitol (5%), Sorbitol (5%), Xylitol (5%) and Polysorbate 80 (0.5%)	Ibuprofen, Cimitedine, Vitamine C, Calcium carbonate/Vitamine D or Acetaminophen
Sucrose (84.75%), Sorbitol (12%), α – Lactose (3%) and Tween 80 (0.25%)	Ibuprofen, Aspirin, Acetaminophen

This process is so named as it utilizes a unique spinning mechanism to produce floss like crystalline structure which mimics cotton candy. This process involves formation of matrix of polysaccharide or saccharide by simultaneous action of flash melting and spinning. The matrix formed is partially recrystallized to have improved flow property and compressibility. This candy floss matrix is then milled and blended with active ingredients and excipients and subsequently compressed in to an ODT. This process can accommodate high dose of drug and offers improved mechanical strength, however high process temperature limits the use of this process to thermo stable compounds only (Bhatu et al., 2011).

The FLASHDOSE is a MDDDS manufactured using Shearform technology in association with Ceform TI™ technology to eliminate the bitter taste of the medicament. The

Shearform technology is employed in the preparation of a matrix known as 'floss', made from a combination of excipients, either alone or with drugs. The floss is a fibrous material similar to cotton-candy fibers, commonly made of saccharides such assucrose, dextrose, lactose and fructose at temperatures ranging between 180–266 °F. However, other polysaccharides such as polymaltodextrins and polydextrose can be transformed into fibers at 30–40% lower temperature than sucrose. This modification permits the safe incorporation of thermo labile drugs into the formulation. The tablets manufactured by this process are highly porous in nature and offer very pleasant mouth feel due to fast solubilization of sugars in presence of saliva.

1.2.9. Direct Compression:

Direct compression is the easiest way to manufacture tablets and ODTs. The great advantage of direct compression is low manufacturing cost. It uses conventional equipment, commonly available excipients and a limited number of processing steps are involved in direct compression. Moreover high doses can be accommodated and final weight of tablet can easily exceed that of other production methods (Dobetti et al., 2001).

The direct compression tablet's disintegration and solubilization are based on the single or combined action of disintegrants, water-soluble excipients, and effervescent agents. The disintegration time is, in general, satisfactory, although the disintegrating efficacy is strongly affected by tablet size and hardness. Large, hard tablets can have a disintegration time greater than that usually required for ODTs. As a consequence, products with optimal disintegration properties often have a medium-small size (weight) and/or a low physical resistance (high friability and low hardness) are formulated but breakage of tablet edges during handling, the presence of deleterious powder in the blistering phase, and tablet rupture during the opening of the blister alveolus, all result from insufficient physical resistance (Dobetti et al., 2001).

In many cases the disintegrants have a major role in the disintegration and dissolution process of ODTs made by direct compression. The choice of a suitable type and an optimal amount of disintegrants is paramount for ensuring a high disintegration rate. The addition of other formulation components such as water soluble excipients or effervescent agents can fursther enhance dissolution or disintegration properties. The understanding of disintegrant properties and their effect on formulation has significantly advanced during the last few years, particularly regarding so called super disintegrants.

This technique can now be applied to preparation of ODT because of the availability of improved excipients especially superdisintegrants and sugar based excipients.

(a) Superdisintegrants: In many orally disintegrating tablet technologies based on direct compression, the addition of superdisintegrants principally affects the rate of disintegration and hence the dissolution. The presence of other formulation ingredients such as water-soluble excipients and effervescent agents further hastens the process of disintegration.

(b) Sugar Based Excipients:

This is another approach to manufacture ODT by direct compression. The use of sugar based excipients especially bulking agents like dextrose, fructose, isomalt, lactilol, maltilol, maltose, mannitol, sorbitol, starch hydrolysate, polydextrose and xylitol, which display high aqueous solubility and sweetness, and hence impart taste masking property and a pleasing mouthfeel. Mizumito et al have classified sugar-based excipients into two types on the basis of molding and dissolution rate. Type 1 saccharides (lactose and mannitol) exhibit low mouldability but high dissolution rate. Type 2 saccharides (maltose and maltilol) exhibit high mouldability and low dissolution rate (Debjit et al., 2009).

1.2.10. Nanonization:

A recently developed Nanomelt technology involves reduction in the particle size of drug to nanosize by milling the drug using a proprietary wet-milling technique. The nanocrystals of the drug are stabilized against agglomeration by surface adsorption on selected stabilizers, which are then incorporated into ODTs. This technique is especially advantageous for poorly water soluble drugs (Gupta et al., 2010). Other advantages of this technology include fast disintegration/dissolution of nanoparticles leading to increased absorption and hence higher bioavailability and reduction in dose, cost effective manufacturing process, conventional packaging due to exceptional durability and wide range of doses (up to 200 mg of drug per unit).

1.2.11. Effervescent method:

Orodispersible tablets are also prepared by effervescent method by mixing sodium bicarbonate and tartaric acid of concentration 12% (w/w) along with super disintegrants like pregelatinized starch, sodium starch glycolate, crospovidone, and croscarmellose. First, sodium bicarbonate and tartaric acid were preheated at a temperature of 80°C to remove absorbed/residual moisture and thoroughly mixed in the motor. Finally, the blends are compressed in the punch.

The major advantages of this method are it is well established, easy to implement and mask the bitter taste of the drug. The effervescent system is generally composed of a dry acid and dry base which when react facilitate a mild effervescent action when the tablet contact with saliva. The effervescent reaction accelerates the disintegration of tablet through the release of carbon dioxide, water and salt. Due to the evolution of Carbon dioxide, the bitter taste of the drug is also masked and a pleasant mouth feel is felt. The major drawbacks of these methods includes chemical stability for which controlled humidity conditions required and storage conditions like temperature and hygroscopicity.

1.3. Patented technologies for oral disintegrating tablets:

Each technology has a different mechanism, and each fast-dissolving/ disintegrating dosage form varies regarding the following.

- Mechanical strength of final product
- Drug and dosage form stability
- Mouth feel
- Taste
- Rate of dissolution of drug formulation in saliva
- Swallow ability
- Rate of absorption from the saliva solution and
- Overall bioavailability.

The various technologies are developed for the preparation of orally disintegrating drug delivery system that are:

1. Zydis
2. Lyoc
3. Orasolv
4. Durasolv
5. Wow tab
6. Flashtab
7. Frosta
8. Advatab
9. Flash dose
10. Oraquick
11. Nanocrystal

12. Pharmaburst
13. Fast melt
14. Multi flash

1.3.1. Zydis:

Zydis is a patented technology by R.P. Scherer. This technology includes physical trapping of the drug in a matrix composed of a Saccharides and a polymer. Zydis, the best known of the fast-dissolving/disintegrating tablet preparations, was the first marketed new technology tablet. 'Zydis' is the first mouth dissolving dosage form in the market. It is a unique freeze-dried tablet in which the active drug is incorporated in a water-soluble matrix, which is then transformed into blister pockets and freeze dried to remove water by sublimation. Zydis matrix is made up of a number of ingredients in order to obtain different objectives. Polymers such as gelatin, dextran or alginates are added to impart strength during handling. These form a glossy and amorphous structure. Mannitol or sorbitol is added to impart crystallinity, elegance and hardness. Various gums may be added to prevent sedimentation of dispersed drug particles. Water is used as a medium to ensure the formation of a porous dosage form. Collapse protectants like glycine may be used to prevent shrinkage of dosage form during freeze drying and long term storage. If necessary, suspending agents and pH adjusting agents may be used. Preservatives may also be added to prevent microbial growth. Zydis products are packed in blister packs to protect the formulation from environmental moisture. A secondary moisture proof foil punch is often required as this dosage form is very moisture sensitive. When put into the mouth, Zydis unit quickly disintegrates and dissolves in saliva (Rosie et al., 2009).

The amount of drug that could be incorporated should generally be less than 60mg for soluble drugs. The particle size of the insoluble drugs should be less than 50 mm and not more than 200 mm to prevent sedimentation during processing. There are some disadvantages to the Zydis technology. The process of freeze-drying is a relatively expensive manufacturing process. The Zydis formulation is very lightweight and fragile, and therefore should not be stored in backpacks or the bottom of purses. Finally, the Zydis formulation has poor stability at higher temperatures and humidities. It readily absorbs water, and is very sensitive to degradation at humidities greater than 65%.

1.3.2. Lyoc

Lyoc is a patented technology of 'PHARMALYOC' (now Cephalon). Lyoc is a porous, solid wafer manufactured by lyophilizing oil in water emulsion placed directly in a blister and subsequently sealed (Shukla et al., 2009). Non homogeneity during freeze drying is avoided by incorporating inert filler (mannitol) to increase the viscosity of the in process suspension. The high proportion of filler reduces the porosity of the tablets due to which disintegration is lowered. The wafers can accommodate high drug dosing and disintegrates rapidly but has poor mechanical strength and non homogeneity during freeze.

1.3.3. Orasolv Technology:

Orasolv was Cima's first fast-dissolving/disintegrating dosage form. The Orasolv technology, unlike Zydis, disperses in the saliva with the aid of almost imperceptible effervescence. An essential feature of this technology is presence of "effervescent couple" that acts as disintegrating agent, while at the same time assisting with taste masking and providing a pleasant "fizzing" sensation in mouth. Concentration of effervescent mixture usually employed is 20 – 25% of tablet weight (Yourong et al., 2004). The Orasolv technology is best described as a fast disintegrating tablet; the tablet matrix dissolves in less than one minute, leaving coated drug powder. The taste masking associated with the Orasolv formulation is two-fold. The unpleasant flavor of a drug is not merely counteracted by sweeteners or flavors; both coating the drug powder and effervescence are means of taste masking in Orasolv. This technology is frequently used to develop over-the-counter formulations. The major disadvantage of the Orasolv formulations is its mechanical strength. The Orasolv tablet has the appearance of a traditional compressed tablet. However, the Orasolv tablets are only lightly compressed, yielding a weaker and more brittle tablet in comparison with conventional tablets.

For that reason, Cima developed a special handling and packaging system for Orasolv. An advantage that goes along with the low degree of compaction of Orasolv is that the particle coating used for taste masking is not compromised by fracture during processing (Manoj et al., 2010). Lyophilization and high degrees of compression, as utilized in Orasolv's primary competitors, may disrupt such as taste masking approach. The Orasolv technology is utilized in six marketed products. These formulations can accommodate single or multiple active ingredients and tablets containing more that 1.0 g of drug have been developed. Their disintegration time is less than 30 sec. The Orasolv formulations are not very hygroscopic.

The Orasolv tablets are soft and fragile in nature, thus a special packaging called 'Paksolv' is needed to protect tablets from breaking during storage and transport. 'Paksolv' is a dome shaped blister package which prevents vertical movement of tablets within the depression. 'Paksolv' offers moisture, light and child resistant packaging.

1.3.4. Durasolv Technology:

Durasolv is Cima's second generation fast-dissolving/disintegrating tablet formulation. Produced in a fashion similar to Orasolv, Durasolv has much higher mechanical strength than its predecessor due to the use of higher compaction pressures during tableting. Durasolv tablets are prepared by using conventional tabletting equipment and have good rigidity (friability less than that 2%). The Durasolv product is thus produced in a faster and more cost-effective manner. Durasolv is so durable that it can be packaged in either traditional blister packaging pouches, vials (Manoj et al, 2010).

One disadvantage of Durasolv is that the technology is not compatible with larger doses of active ingredients, because the formulation is subjected to such high pressures on compaction. Unlike Orasolv, the structural integrity of any taste masking may be compromised with high drug doses. The drug powder coating in Durasolv may become fractured during compaction, exposing the bitter-tasting drug to a patient's taste buds. Therefore the Durasolv technology is best suited for formulations including relatively small doses of active compound.

1.3.5. Wow tab Technology:

The Wowtab fast-dissolving/disintegrating tablet formulation has been on the Japanese market for a number of years. Wowtab technology is patented by Yamanouchi Pharmaceutical. The WOW in Wowtab signifies the tablet is to be given "Without Water". It has just recently been introduced into the U.S. The Wowtab technology utilizes sugar and sugar-like (e.g., mannitol) excipients.

This process uses a combination of low mouldability saccharides (eg. lactose, glucose, sucrose, xylitol and mannitol) which shows rapid dissolution and high mouldability saccharide (eg. Multitol, maltose, sorbitol and oligosaccharides) which shows good binding property (Kuchekar et al., 2003). The two different types of saccharides are combined to obtain a tablet formulation with adequate hardness and fast dissolution rate. Due to its significant hardness, the Wowtab formulation is a bit more stable to the environment than the

Zydis or OraSolv. It is suitable for both conventional bottle and blister packaging. The taste masking technology utilized in the Wowtab is proprietary, but claims to offer superior mouth feel due to the patented SMOOTHMELT action. The Wowtab product dissolves quickly in 15 seconds.

1.3.6. Flashtab Technology:

Prographarm laboratories have patented the Flashtab technology. This technology involves the preparation of rapidly disintegrating tablet which consists of an active ingredient in the form of microcrystals. Drug microgranules may be prepared by using the conventional techniques like coacervation, extrusion-spheronization, simple pan coating methods and microencapsulation.

The microcrystals of microgranules of the active ingredient are added to the granulated mixture of excipients prepared by wet or dry granulation, and compressed into tablets. All the processing utilized the conventional tabletting technology, and the tablets produced are reported to have good mechanical strength and disintegration time less than one minute (Rosie et al., 2009).

1.3.7. Frosta technology:

Akina patents this technology. It utilizes the concept of formulating plastic granules and compressing them at low pressure to produce strong tablets with high porosity. Plastic granules composed of porous and plastic material, water penetration enhancer, and binder. The process involves mixing the porous plastic material with water penetration enhancer followed by granulating with binder. The tablets obtained have excellent hardness and rapid disintegration time ranging from 15 to 30 sec depending on size of tablet (Seong et al., 2008).

1.3.8. Advatab:

Eurand is the owner of advatab drug delivery system. Eurand is known for its microcaps technology, which involves taste masking drug particles using microencapsulation process based on coacervation technique to mask the taste along with restriction of drug dissolution in the mouth cavity. The primary ingredients in the dosage form include sugar alcohols and saccharide with particle size less than 30mm along with disintegrant and lubricant. Advatab tablets disintegrate rapidly in mouth, typically in less than 30s, to allow for convenient oral drug administration without water. These tablets can be packed both bottles and pushed through blisters (Debjit et al., 2009).

1.3.9. Flash dose:

Fuisz Technologies has three oral drug delivery systems that are related to fast dissolution. The first two generations of quick-dissolving tablets, Soft Chew and EZ Chew, require some chewing. However, these paved the way for Fuisz's most recent development, Flash Dose (Rajan et al., 2001). The Flash Dose technology utilizes a unique spinning mechanism to produce a floss-like crystalline structure, much like cotton candy. This crystalline sugar can then incorporate the active drug and be compressed into a tablet. This procedure has been patented by Fuisz and is known as Shearform.The final product has a very high surface area for dissolution. It disperses and dissolves quickly once placed onto the tongue.

Flash dose tablets consists of self-binding shear form matrix termed as "floss". Shear form matrices are prepared by flash heat processing and are of two types.

- Single floss or Unifloss, consisting of a carrier, and two or more sugar alcohols, of which one is xylitol.
- Dual floss consists of a first shear form carrier material (termed 'base floss', contains a carrier and at least one sugar alcohol generally sorbitol), and a second shear form binder matrix ('binder floss', contains a carrier and xylitol).

Interestingly, by changing the temperature and other conditions during production, the characteristics of the product can be altered greatly. Instead of a floss-like material, small spheres of saccharides can be produced to carry the drug. The process of making microspheres has been patented by Fuisz, and is known as CEFORM and serves as an alternative method of taste masking.

1.3.10. Oraquick Technology:

The Oraquick fast-dissolving/disintegrating tablet formulation utilizes a patented taste masking technology. KV Pharmaceutical claims its microsphere technology, known as MicroMask, has superior mouth feel over taste-masking alternatives. The taste masking process does not utilize solvents of any kind, and therefore leads to faster and more efficient production. Also, lower heat of production than alternative fast-dissolving/disintegrating technologies makes Oraquick appropriate for heat-sensitive drugs. KV Pharmaceutical also claims that the matrix that surrounds and protects the drug powder in microencapsulated particles is more pliable, meaning tablets can be compressed to achieve significant mechanical strength without disrupting taste masking.

Oraquick claims quick dissolution in a matter of seconds, with good taste-masking. There are no products using the Oraquick technology currently on the market, but KV Pharmaceutical has products in development such as analgesics, scheduled drugs, cough and cold, psycho tropics, and anti -infectiveS (Manoj et al., 2010).

1.3.11. Nanocrystal Technology:

For oral disintegrating tablets, Élan's proprietary Nanocrystal technology can enable formulation and improve compound activity and final product characteristics. Decreasing particle size increases the surface area, which leads to an increase in dissolution rate. This can be accomplished predictably and efficiently using Nanocrystal technology (Yourong et al., 2004). Nanocrystal particles are small particles of drug substance, typically less than 1000 nanometers (nm) in diameter, which are produced by milling the drug substance using a proprietary wet milling technique.

Nanocrystal fast dissolving technology provides for:

- Pharmacokinetic benefits of orally administered Nanoparticles (<2 microns) in the form of a rapidly disintegrating tablet matrix.
- Product differentiation based upon a combination of proprietary and patent-protected technology elements.
- Cost-effective manufacturing processes that utilize conventional, scalable unit operations.
- Exceptional durability, enabling use of conventional packaging equipment and formats (i.e., bottles and/or blisters).
- Wide range of doses (up to 200mg of API per unit).
- Use of conventional, compendial inactive components.
- Employment of non-moisture sensitive inactives.

Nanocrystal colloidal dispersions of drug substance are combined with water-soluble GRAS (Generally Regarded as Safe) ingredients, filled into blisters, and lyophilized. The resultant wafers are remarkably robust, yet dissolve in very small quantities of water in seconds. This approach is especially attractive when working with highly potent or hazardous materials because it avoids manufacturing operations (e.g., granulation, blending, and tableting) that generate large quantities of aerosolized powder and present much higher risk of exposure. The freeze-drying approach also enables small quantities of drug to be converted into ODT dosage forms because manufacturing losses are negligible.

1.3.12. Pharmaburst:

This is a patented technology of SPI Pharma. New castle. It utilizes the concept of co-processed excipients to develop ODT which dissolves within 30-4 seconds. This technology involves dry blending of drug, flavor and lubricant followed by compression into tablets. Tablets manufactured by this process sufficient strength, so they can be packed in blister packs (Madhusudan Rao et al., 2010).

1.3.13. Fast melt:

It is a patented technology of Elan Corporation. It forms highly porous, microfine matrix tablets which once placed on tongue; the matrix rapidly absorbs water and disintegrates. The drug is in a stabilized, size reduced form to ensure optimal solubility which dissolves rapidly. The combination of mild effervescent base and drug processing ensures that the dosage form goes into solution in 15-30 seconds.

1.3.14. Multiflash:

Multiflash is a multi unit tablet composed of coated microgranules and fast disintegrating excipients. This multi particulate tablet quickly disintegrates in the esophagus after being swallowed with a minimum amount of water. This tablet avoids mucosal adhesion and coated pellets can match various dissolution rates (Rajan et al., 2001).

1.4. Role of super disintegrants in odts

The basic approach in development of ODTs is use of disintegrant. Disintegrant plays as important role in the disintegration and dissolution of ODT. It is essential to choose a suitable disintegrant, in an optimum concentration so as to ensure quick disintegration and high dissolution rates.

Superdisintegrant provide quick disintegration due to combined effect of swelling and water absorption by the formulation. Due to swelling of superdisintegrant, the wetted surface of the carrier increases; this promotes the wetability and dispersibility of the system, thus enhancing the disintegration and dissolution.

Care should be taken to taken while selecting concentration of the superdisintegrant. Superdisintegrants are selected according to critical concentration of disintegrant. Below this concentration, the tablet disintegration time is inversely proportional to the concentration of the superdisintegrant, whereas if concentration of super disintegrant is above critical concentration, the disintegration time remains almost constant or even increases.

Common disintegrants used in this formulation are croscarmellose sodium (Vivasol, Ac-Di-Sol), crospovidone (Polyplasdone), carmellose (NS-300), carmellose calcium (ECG-505), sodium starch glycolate (SSG) etc. Recently few ion exchange resins (e.g. Indion 414) are found to have super-disintegrant property and are widely used in pharmaceutical industry.

1.5. Mechanism of Super disintegrants:

There are major mechanisms for tablets disintegration as follows (Khuldeep et al., 2010)

1.5.1. Swelling:

Perhaps the most widely accepted general mechanism of action for tablet disintegration is swelling. Tablets with high porosity show poor disintegration due to lack of adequate swelling force. On the other hand, sufficient swelling force is exerted in the tablet with low porosity. It is worthwhile to note that if the packing fraction is very high, fluid is unable to penetrate in the tablet and disintegration is again slows down.

1.5.2. Porosity and capillary action (Wicking) :

Disintegration by capillary action is always the first step. When we put the tablet into suitable aqueous medium, the medium penetrates into the tablet and replaces the air adsorbed on the particles, which weakens the intermolecular bond and breaks the tablet into fine particles. Water uptake by tablet depends upon hydrophilicity of the drug /excipient and on tableting conditions.

For these types of disintegrants maintenance of porous structure and low interfacial tension towards aqueous fluid is necessary which helps in disintegration by creating a hydrophilic network around the drug particles (Debjit et al., 2009).

WICKING	SWELLING
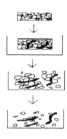	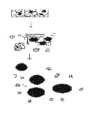
Disintegrant pulls water into the pores and reduces the physical bonding forces between particles	Particles swell and break up the matrix from within; swelling sets up; localized stress spreads throughout the matrix

Figure 2. Disintegration of tablet by wicking and swelling

1.5.3. Due to disintegrating particle/particle repulsive forces:

Another mechanism of disintegration attempts to explain the swelling of tablet made with 'nonswellable' disintegrants. Guyot-Hermann has proposed a particle repulsion theory based on the observation that nonswelling particle also cause disintegration of tablets. The electric repulsive forces between particles are the mechanism of disintegration and water is required for it. Researchers found that repulsion is secondary to wicking (Tejvir et al., 2011).

1.5.4. Due to deformation:

During tablet compression, disintegrated particles get deformed and these deformed particles get into their normal structure when they come in contact with aqueous media or water. Occasionally, the swelling capacity of starch was improved when granules were extensively deformed during compression. This increase in size of the deformed particles produces a breakup of the tablet. This may be a mechanism of starch and has only recently begun to be studied.

DEFORMATION	REPULSION
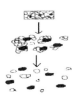	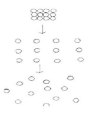
Particles swell to pre compression size and break up matrix	Water is drawn into pores and particles repel each other because of resulting electrical force.

Figure 3. Disintegration of tablet by deformation and repulsion

1.5.5. Because of heat of wetting (air expansion):

When disintegrantes with exothermic properties gets wetted, localized stress is generated due to capillary air expansion, which helps in disintegration of tablet. This explanation, however, is limited to only a few types of disintegrants and cannot describe the action of most modern disintegrating agents (Tejvir et al 2011).

1.5.6. Due to release of gases :

Carbon dioxide released within tablets on wetting due to interaction between bicarbonate and carbonate with citric acid or tartaric acid. The tablet disintegrates due to generation of pressure within the tablet. This effervescent mixture is used when pharmacist needs to formulate very rapidly dissolving tablets or fast disintegrating tablet.

As these disintegrants are highly sensitive to small changes in humidity level and temperature, strict control of environment is required during manufacturing of the tablets. The effervescent blend is either added immediately prior to compression or can be added in to two separate fraction of formulation.

1.5.7. By enzymatic reaction :

Here, enzymes present in the body act as disintegrants. These enzymes destroy the binding action of binder and helps in disintegration. Actually due to swelling, pressure exerted in the outer direction or radial direction, it causes tablet to burst or the accelerated absorption of water leading to an enormous increase in the volume of granules to promote disintegration

Table 2. oral disintegrating tablets currently available in market

Product	Manufactured By/For	Active ingredient	Category	Indication	Intended Age Group
Abilify Discmelt	Otsuka America/Bristol-Myers Squibb	aripiprazole	Atypical antipsychotics	Schizophrenia Bipolar disorder, adjunct therapy for Major Depressive Disorder	13 years+ for Schizophrenia, 10 years+ for Bipolar disorder, adults for MDD.
Alavert Quick Dissolving Tablets	Wyeth	Loratadine	Anti-histamines	Allergy	6 years+
Allegra ODT	Sanofi Aventis	Fexofenadine	Anti-histamines	Allergic rhinitis, Urticaria	6-11 years
Aricept ODT	Eisai Co.	Donepezil	Acetylcholinesterase inhibitors	Alzheimer's disease	Adults
Benadryl FastMelt	Pfizer	Diphenhydramine	Anti-histamines	Allergy	6 years+
Calpol Fast Melts	McNeil Healthcare UK	Paracetamol	Analgesics	Pain	6 years+
Clarinex RediTabs	Schering-Plough	Desloratadine	Anti-histamines	Allergy	6 years+
Claritin RediTabs	Schering-Plough	Loratadine	Anti-histamines	Allergy	6 years+
Clonazepam ODT	Par Pharmaceuticals	Clonazepam	Benzodiazepin-es	Anxiety, Panic Disorder, Seizure Disorders	infants+
Product	Manufactured By	Active ingredient	Category	Indication	Intended Age Group

Fazaclo	Azurpharma	Clozapine	Anti-psycho-tics	Treatment resistant schizophrenia	Adults
Klonopin Wafers	Roche	Clonazepam	Benzodiazepi-nes	Panic Disorder, Seizure Disorders	infants+ for seizure disorders, adults for Panic Disorder
Lamictal ODT	Eurand/ Glaxo Smith Kline	lamotrigine	Anti-convulsant	Bipolar Disorter, Epilepsy	18+ for bipolar, 2+ for seizure
Loratadine Redidose	Ranbaxy	loratadine	Anti- histamines	Allergy	6 years+

DRUG PROFILE

Drug : Tolterodine tartrate

Drug category : Tolterodine tartrate is a new competitive muscarinic receptor antagonist used in the treatment of overactive bladder with symptoms of urinary frequency.

Brand name : Detrol - LA

IUPAC name : (R)-N, N- di isopropyl -3-(2-hydroxy-5-methylphenyl)-3-phenylpropanamine L-hydrogen tartrate

Chemical formula : $C_{26}H_{37}NO_7$

Molecular weight : 475.06

BCS class	:	Class I
Sructure	:	

PHYSICOCHEMICAL PROPERTIES:

Description	:	White, crystalline powder.
Solubility	:	Practically insoluble in toluene and sparingly soluble in Water soluble in methanol, and slightly soluble in ethanol
Melting point	:	205-210^{0}C

PHARMACOKINETIC PROPETIES:

Oral bioavailability	: 77 %.
Plasma half life	: 1.9-3.7hours.
Absorption	: Absorbed its maximum serum concentration 1-2 hours
Metabolism	: Metabolised by the liver
Elimination	: Elimination by urine
Therapeutical category	: Anti cholinergic Agents
Mechanism of action	: Tolterodine act on M1, M2, M, M4 and M5 subtypes of muscarinic receptor, where as modern anti muscarinic treatments for over active bladder only act on M3.
Therapeutic/clinical use	: Tolteridone Tartrate is a new competitive muscarinic receptor antagonist used in the treatment of overactive bladder with symptoms of urinary frequency, urgency, and incontinence.

Adverse effects:

- Hypo salivation
- Dry eyes
- Decreased gastric motility
- Constipation
- Headache
- Slepiness

Contraindications : Tolterodine is contraindicated in patients with urinary retention, gastric retention, or uncontrolled narrow angle glaucoma, hepatic impairment and hyper sensitivity to the drug or its ingredients.

Table 3. Drug Interactions

Drug	Interaction
Fluaxetine	Significantly inhibited the metabolism of Tolterodine, in extensive metaboliser, resulting in 4.8-Fold increased in Tolterodine AUC, decreased in C max
Warfarine	Increases the effect and toxicity of Tolterodine Tartrate
Ethinyl oestadiol	Possible loss of contraceptive effect
Levonorgesterl	Pssible loss of contraceptive effect
Hydrochlorothiazide	Increases the effect and toxicity of Tolterodine Tartrate
Erythromycine	Increases the toxicity of Tolterodine Tartrate
Miconazole, Ketoconazole	Increases the effect and toxicity of Tolterodine Tartrate
Tricyclic anti depresants	Tolterodine may influence the pharmacokinetics of drugs that are metabolized by P450 2D6 such as tri cyclic anti depressents

Table 4. Dosage form and dose

Route	Dosage forms	Strength
Oral	Tablets	2 mg
	Tablets	4mg
	Tablets	6mg

2. METHODOLOGY

2.1. Preparation of standard graph of Tolterodine Tartrate in 0.1NHCl

Accurately weighed amount (100mg) of the drug was dissolved in 0.1NHCl in 100mL volumetric flask and make up the volume to 100mL with 0.1N HCl. Form this stock solution (1mg/mL) 10mL of solution is with drawn into a 100mL volumetric flask and the volume was made up with 0.1NHCl. Form this second solution (100µg/mL) different concentration 5, 10, 20, 25, 30, 35, 40 and 45 µg/mL are prepared and their corresponding absorbance was measured at 216 nm in a UV/Visible spectrophotometer.

2.2. Preparation of standard graph of Tolterodine Tartrate in pH 6.8 Phoshpate buffer

Accurately weighed amount (100mg) of the drug was dissolved was dissolved in 50mL solvent mixture of phosphate buffer (pH 6.8) which constitutes the stock solution of 1 mg/mL. Form this stock solution (1mg/mL) 10mL of solution is with drawn into a 100mL volumetric flask and the volume was made up with pH 6.8 phosphate buffer. Form this second solution (100µg/mL) different concentration 5, 10, 15, 20, 25, 30, and 35 µg/mL are prepared and their corresponding absorbance was measured at 216 nm in a UV/Visible spectrophotometer.

2.3. Preparation of Drug - Polymer Complex

Tolterodine Tartrate and EudragitEPO complex was prepared by solvent evaporation method. Saturated stock solutions of Tolterodine Tartrate and Eudragit EPO were prepared in absolute Ethanol. Aliquots of drug and polymer solutions were taken to obtain various ratios (1:1, 1:2 and 1:3,) and mixed continuously at 150rpm on a magnetic stirrer. Stirring was allowed to continue until the solvent is completely evaporated (Shagufta et al., 2007). After this mixture was kept at 35°C for 2 hours and dried at room temperature for 24 hours to obtain a hard matrix. Then the hard matrix is subsequently pulverized and screened through 60mesh to obtain the uniform sized fine powder of drug polymer complex (DPC) and it was finally stored in a tightly closed container for further studies.

General formula : A formula is set using following ingredients

Drug	Tolterodine Tartrate
Disintegrants	Crosspovidone / Croscarmellose sodium / Sodium starch glycolate
Bulking agent	Microcrystalline cellulose
Sweetening agent	Sodium saccharine
Flavoring agent	Orange
Lubricant	Sodium stearylfumarate
Glidant	Aerosil

Total tablet weight was set to be 80 mg punch size is set to be 5mm

2.4. Preparation of Tolterodine Tartrate ODTs by direct compression technique

Tolterodine Tartrate ODTs were prepared using direct compression technique. Direct compression technique is a convenient method. Different formulations of TolterodineTartrate ODTs were designed to be prepared by direct compression technique using four super disintegrants, (Crosspovidone, Croscarmellosesodium, and Sodium starch glycolate). Superdisintegrants is varied with 3 different concentrations (i.e., 4, 6 and 8% respectively) keeping all other ingredients constant, there are assigned with formulation codes shown in Table 5.

Table 5. Formulation codes of ODTs

Disintegrant used	Concentration (%)	Formulation code
Crosspovidone	4 6 8	F1 F2 F3
Crosscarmellose Sodium	4 6 8	F4 F5 F6
Sodium starch glycolate	4 6 8	F7 F8 F9
Crosspovidone + Sodium starch glycolate	4 6 8	F10 F11 F12
Crosspovidone + Crosscarmelose sodium	4 6 8	F13 F14 F15
Crosscarmellosesodiums + Sodium starch glycolate	4 6 8	F16 F17 F18

Procedure:

Drug-Polymer complex, superdisintegrants, microcrystalline cellulose, sodium saccharine, orange flavor were accurately weighed and passed through a 40-mesh screen to get uniform size particles and mixed in a glass mortar for 15 minutes. The obtained blend was lubricated with sodium stearylfumarate and aerosil and mixing was continued for further 5 minutes. The resultant mixture was directly compressed into tablets by using 5mm round concave faced punch of Rotary tabletting machine. Compression force was kept constant for all formulations. Table 3.3 outlines the compositions of various ODT formulations.

Table 6. Formulation of TolterodineTattrate ODTs preparedby direct compression method with various superdisintegrants

Ingredients	Super disintegrants concentration (%) of Crosspovidone/ Croscarmellose Sodium/ Sodium starch glycolate		
	4%	6%	8%
Drug-Polymer complex(1:2)	12	12	12
Pearlitol SD 200	8	8	8
Avicel pH 102	52	50.4	48.8
Super disintegrants	3.2	4.8	6.4
Sodium saccharine (2%)	1.6	1.6	1.6
Orange flavor (2%)	1.6	1.6	1.6
Sodium stearylfumarate (0.25%)	0.8	0.8	0.8
Aerosil	0.8	0.8	0.8

2.5. Evaluation of DPC drug content and *in-Vitro* taste evaluation

Drug content was determined by dissolving 100mg of DPC in100mL of simulated gastric fluid (SGF) and analyzing diluted sample at 216nm by UV- spectrophotometer. *In Vitro* taste was evaluated by determining drug release in simulated salivary fluid (SSF) (pH6.8) to predict drug release in human saliva. DPC, equivalent to 4mg of Tolterodine Tartrate, its dose, was placed in 10mL of SSF and shaken for 60 seconds. The amount of drug released was analyzed at 216nm by UV-spectrophotometer.

2.6. Evaluation of orally disintegration tablet formulations:

Different quality control tests were performed for all the ODTs formulations to check whether these have met the specifications given in USP along with other *in vitro* tests like wetting time and water absorption ratio.

Warious *in vitro* tests performed are:
- Weight variation test

- Thickness measurement
- Hardness and Friability
- Content uniformity
- Wetting time and Water absorption ratio
- Disintegration Time
- Dissolution test

Weight variation test:

Method: Twenty tablets were randomly selected from each formulation and their average weight was calculated by using an electronic balance (Shimadzu, AUX 220, Shimadzu Corp, Japan) Individual weight of each tablet was also calculated using the same and compared with the average weight. The Mean ± S.D. were noted.

Table 7. Weight Variation Limits

IP/BP	Limit	USP
80 mg or less	10%	130mg or less
More than 80mg or Less than 250mg	7.5%	130mg to 324mg
250mg or more	5%	More than 324mg

Thickness measurement

Method: Randomly ten tablets were taken from each formulation and their thickness was measured using a digital Verniercaliper (Mitutoyo Corp, Kawasaki, Japan). Average thickness and standard deviation values were calculated. The tablet thickness should be controlled within a ± 5% variation of standard value.

Hardness

Method: The tablet hardness of different formulations was measured using the Monsanto hardness tester. The tester consists of a barrel containing a compressible spring held between two plungers. The lower plunger was placed in contact with the tablet, and a zero was taken. The upper plunger was then forced against the spring by turning a threaded bolt until the tablet fractures. As the spring is compressed, a pointer rides along a gauge in the barrel to indicate the force. The force of fracture is recorded, and the zero force reading is deducted from it. Generally, a minimum hardness of 4 kg is considered acceptable for uncoated tablets. The hardness for ODTs should be preferably 1-3 kg.

Friability

Method: This test is performed using a laboratory friability tester known as Roche Friabilator. Ten tablets were weighed and placed in a plastic chambered friabilator attached to a motor, which revolves at a speed of 25 rpm, dropping the tablets from a distance of 6 inches with each revolution. The tablets were subjected to 100 revolutions for 4 minutes. After the process, these tablets were dedusted and reweighed. Percentage loss of tablet weight was calculated.

$$\% \text{ Friability} = (W_1 - W_2) \times 100/W_1$$

Where,

W_1 = Initial weight of the 10 tablets.

W_2 = Final weight of the 10 tablets.

Friability values below 1% are generally acceptable.

Content uniformity:

Ten tablets were randomly selected, weighed and finely powdered and quantity of powder equivalent to one tablet was added to 100ml 0.1N HCl in a conical flask. Conical flasks were placed on a rotary shaker. An aliquot of solution was centrifuged and supernatant was filtered through a 0.22µ filter. Absorbance of the resulted supernatant solution was measured using UV Visible spectrophotometer at a wavelength of 216nm against 0.1N HCl as blank. Concentrations were calculated with the help of standard graph and total amount present in the formulation was calculated.

Wetting time:

A piece of tissue paper folded twice was placed in a small petridish containing 6ml of water. A water-soluble dyephenolphthalein was added to the petri dish. The dye solution is used to identify the complete wetting of the tablet surface(Abdelbary et al, 2009). A tablet was carefully placed on the surface of tissue paper in the petri dish at room temperature. The time required for water to reach the upper surface of the tablets and completely wet them was noted as the wetting time. To check for reproducibility, the measurements were carried out in replicates (n=6). The wetting time was recorded using a stopwatch.

Water absorption ratio (R):

The weight of the tablet before keeping in the petri dish was noted (W_b) using Shimadzu digital balance. The wetted tablet from the petri dish was taken and reweighed (W_a) using the same. The Water absorption ratio, R, was determined according to the following equation:

$R = 100 (W_a - W_b) / W_b$

Where W_b and W_a are the weight before and after water absorption respectively.

Disintegration time:

Disintegration time is considered to be one of the important criteria in selecting the best formulation. *In-vitro* disintegration time for ODTs was determined by using USP disintegration apparatus type II (Paddle) (Electrolab ED-2L, India) with 6.8pH phosphate buffer as the disintegration medium. The medium was maintained at 37±0.5°C (Samprasit et al., 2011). The time point at which tablet completely disintegrates is noted as Disintegration time.

Dissolution test:

Method: Dissolution test was carried out using USP rotating paddle method (apparatus 2). The stirring rate was 50 rpm. 6.8 pH phosphate buffer and methanol (1:1) was used as dissolution medium (900ml) and was maintained at 37 ± 1^0C. Samples of 5mL were withdrawn at predetermined intervals (2, 4, 6, 8, 10, 15, 20, 25 and 30 min), filtered and replaced with 5mL of fresh dissolution medium.

The collected samples were suitably diluted with dissolution fluid, where ever necessary and were analyzed for the Tolterodine Tartrate at 216 nm by using UV spectrophotometer. Each dissolution study was performed for three times and mean values were taken.

In Vivo taste evaluation:

Taste evaluation was conducted on eight healthy human volunteers from whom informed consent was obtained. The Drug-Polymer complex equivalent of 4mg of Tolterodine Tartrate was place on the tongue for 30 seconds and then spat out. Optimized ODT formulation (containing 4 mg of Tolterodine Tartrate) was placed on the tongue until complete disintegration (Jianchen et al., 2008). Taste was evaluated and assigned according to bitterness intensity scale, i.e. 0=tasteless, 1=slight bitter, 2=moderate bitter, 3=strong bitter.

In Vivo disintegration time:

Oral disintegration time of optimized formulation was performed on eight healthy human volunteers from whom informed consent was obtained. Prior to the test all the volunteers were asked to rinse their mouth with the distilled water. Tablets were placed on the tongue and the time required for the complete disintegration of tablets was recorded. Immediately after the disintegration of the tablet, volunteers were asked to rinse their mouth without ingesting disintegrating materials (Goel et al., 2011). This experiment was conducted in eight volunteers

(3 tablets per volunteer) and the mean±SD were calculated for each.

3. RESULTS

3.1. Construction of calibration curve of Tolterodine Tartrate

The calibration curve of Tolterodine Tartrate has shown good linearity with R^2 value 0.998 in 0.1NHCl by plotting concentration on X-axis and absorbance on Y-axis

Table 8. Calibration curve for the estimation of TolterodineTartrate in 0.1NHCl

S.NO	Concentration(µg/mL)	UV-absorbance(n=5)
1	2	0.153±0.005
2	4	0.292±0.09
3	6	0.44±0.012
4	8	0.613±0.018
5	10	0.732±0.006

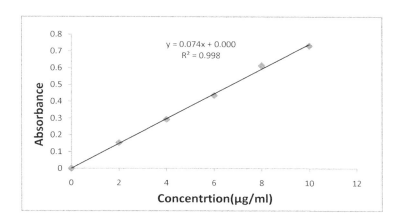

Figure 4. Calibration curve for the estimation of TolterodineTartrate

The calibration curve of Tolterodine Tartrate has shown good linearity with R^2 value 0.997in pH 6.8 phosphatebufferby plotting concentration on X-axis and absorbance on Y-axis

Table 9. Calibration curve for the estimation of Tolterodine Tartrate in pH 6.8 Phosphate buffer:

S.NO	Concentration(µg/mL)	UV-absorbance(n=5)
1	2	0.164±0.003
2	4	0.311±0.05
3	6	0.425±0.09
4	8	0.592±0.015
5	10	0.746±0.007

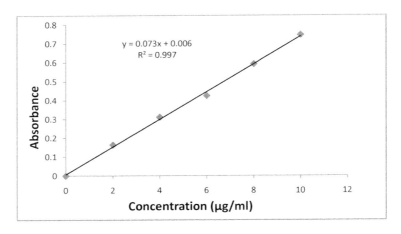

Figure 5. Calibration curve for the estimation of TolterodineTartrate

The present analytical method obeyed Beer's law in the concentration range of 2 – 10 µg/mL and is suitable for the estimation of Tolterodine Tartrate from different solutions. The correlation coefficient (r) value for the linear regression equation was found to be 0.998, in 0.1NHCl and 0.997, inpH 6.8 indicating a positive correlation between the concentration of Tolterodine Tartrate and its corresponding absorbance values.

3.2. Evaluation of DPC Drug content and in-vitro taste evaluation

Percentage drug loading in drug- polymer complex, was found to be 98.15% for 1:2 ratio compared to 1:1 and 1:3 in which drug loading is 92% and 86.7%. No drug release was observed in SSF from complexes with drug-polymer ratio of 1:2 compared to 1:1 and 1:3 ratios, therefore, the ratio 1:2 was considered the optimal DPC with complete taste masking of metallic taste of Tolterodine Tartrate.

Table 10. Evaluation of Drug content and *in-vitro* taste evaluation of DPC

S.No	Drug-Polymer ratio in DPC	Amount of Tolterodine Tartrate per 100 mg of DPC	% Drug Dissolved in SSF
1	1:1	48.51±0.24	7.18±1.07
2	1:2	34.47±0.14	0.33±0.19
3	1:3	24.86±0.5	4.03±0.48

Table 11. Preformulation characteristics of Tolterodine Tartrate ODTs prepared by Varying concentrations of superdisintegrants

Formulation	Bulk density (g/cc)	Tapped density (g/cc)	Hausner ratio	Compressibilty index (%)	Angle of repose
F1	0.379	0.452	1.19	15.55	28.62
F2	0.385	0.465	1.20	14.87	27.20
F3	0.380	0.455	1.19	15.00	25.75
F4	0.392	0.460	1.17	14.55	25.54
F5	0.375	0.445	1.18	14.15	29
F6	0.380	0.447	1.17	15.02	27.42
F7	0.376	0.443	1.17	14.87	27.82
F8	0.372	0.442	1.18	15.31	26.20
F9	0.374	0.439	1.17	15.52	28.35

Table 12. Tabletting characteristics of Tolterodine TartrateODTs

Formulation	Hardness[a] (kg/cm^2)	Friability[b] (%)	Weight[c] (mg)	Thickness[a] (mm)	Drug content[c] (%)
F1	3.2±0.40	0.49	79.90±0.90	3.77±0.02	98.18±0.86
F2	2.46±0.20	0.53	80.07±0.88	3.80±0.01	89.23±1.22
F3	2.78±0.15	0.45	80.10±0.87	3.72±0.02	101.05±1.58
F4	2.88±0.26	0.39	79.73±0.49	3.83±0.07	99.05±0.5
F5	2.73±0.8	0.25	79.89±0.56	3.84±0.09	98.85±1.04
F6	2.52±0.18	0.36	79.99±0.58	3.83±0.01	101.48±0.5
F7	3.2±0.27	0.44	79.96±0.63	3.82±0.02	98.62±0.52
F8	2.96±0.15	0.67	79.83±0.84	3.82±0.01	97.59±0.52
F9	3.5±0.25	0.75	79.54±0.77	3.73±0.01	100.11±1.78

Table 13. Tabletting characteristics of Tolterodine TartrateODTs

Formulation code	Disintegration time[a](sec)	Wetting time[a] (sec)	Water absorption ratio[a]	*In vitro* dispersion time[a] (sec)
F1	44.90±0.92	45.57±0.49	54.21±0.44	45.83±0.88
F2	39.25±0.60	38.07±0.52	62.82±0.18	40.33±0.61
F3	34.16±0.75	32.66±0.54	69.38±0.43	34.21±0.70
F4	32.25±0.76	31.76±0.75	72.16±0.88	32.20±0.60
F5	24.89±0.68	29.74±0.73	89.93±0.20	26.24±0.42
F6	**19.05±0.83**	**23.21±0.67**	**99.89±0.51**	**20.25±0.41**
F7	52.66±1.50	65.74±0.42	37.30±0.46	59.83±0.88
F8	47.22±0.89	51.57±0.49	43.97±0.86	52.83±0.65
F9	45.66±0.81	48.39±0.49	52.88±0.64	46.20±0.50

a: Mean±S.D., n=6 tablets, b: Mean±S.D., n=10, c: Mean±S.D., n=20

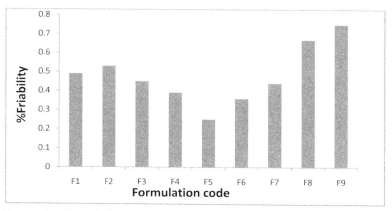

Figure 6. Graphical representation of friability of TolterodineTartrate prepared by varying concentrations of superdisintegrants

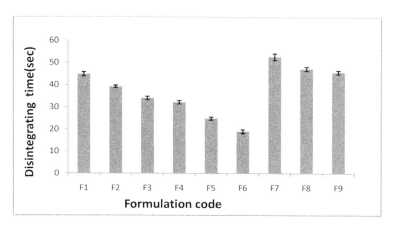

Figure 7. Graphical representation of disintegration times of Tolterodine TartrateODTs prepared by varying concentrations superdisintegrants

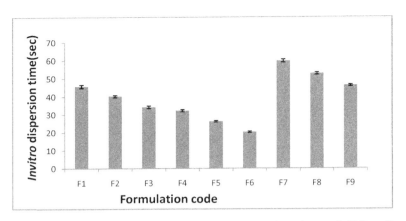

Figure 8. Graphical representation *in vitro* dispersion times of Tolterodine Tartrate ODTs prepared by varying concentrations of superdisintegrants

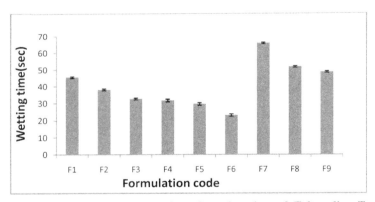

Figure 9. Graphical representation of wetting time of Tolterodine Tartrate ODTs prepared by varying concentrations of superdisintegrants

Table 14. Cumulative percent Tolterodine Tartrate released from ODTs containing varying concentrations of different superdisintegrants

Time (min)	\multicolumn{6}{c}{Cumulative % drug release}					
	F1	F2	F3	F4	F5	F6
2	23.26±0.15	29±0.03	21.33±0.31	22.6±0.22	28.1±0.06	34.55±0.16
4	35.06±0.33	42.7±0.34	36.45±0.66	39.5±0.24	42.2±0.62	49.03±0.45
6	47.07±0.04	53.5±0.16	50.51±0.03	49.2±1.12	52.35±0.25	58.17±1.33
8	59.5±0.48	63.51±0.40	66.12±1.07	56.5±0.62	59.01±0.55	65.42±0.37
10	65.1±1.22	72.76±0.33	69.97±0.22	66.4±0.32	68.02±0.02	71.57±0.02
15	70.96±0.23	81.35±0.05	75.57±0.58	72.5±0.01	76.12±0.57	80.4±0.93
20	82.5±0.40	88.45±0.15	84.23±0.96	82.5±0.92	84.35±0.46	87.21±0.55
25	85.01±0.1	89.64±0.26	89.57±0.13	89.95±0.16	89.45±0.68	93.50±1.42
30	89.8±34.25	90.57±0.44	93.90±0.45	93.88±0.21	95.33±1.27	97.89±0.28

Time (min)	Cumulative % drug release		
	F7	F8	F9
2	20.9±0.22	26.28±0.04	23.42±0.15
4	27.5±0.39	33.48±0.62	34.72±0.28
6	34.94±0.64	40.35±0.48	47.17±0.18
8	49.55±0.46	45.10±0.04	53.92±0.35
10	54.28±0.13	49.29±0.55	57.07±0.99
15	60.69±0.04	60.12±0.36	64.31±0.06
20	64.78±0.47	67.47±0.25	75.32±0.24
25	73.25±0.57	78.25±0.24	82.37±0.26
30	79.89±0.17	83.85±0.52	84.95±0.49

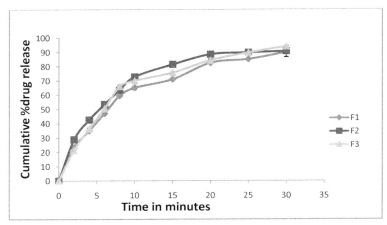

Figure 10. Graphical representation of Cumulative percent Tolterodine Tartrate released from ODTs containing varying concentrations ofcrosspovidone.

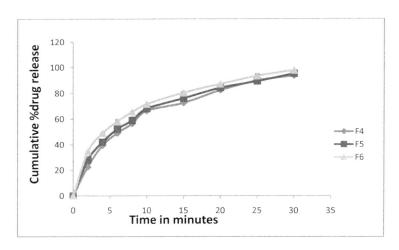

Figure 11. Graphical representation of Cumulative percent Tolterodine Tartrate released from ODTs containing varying concentrations ofcrosscarmelose sodium.

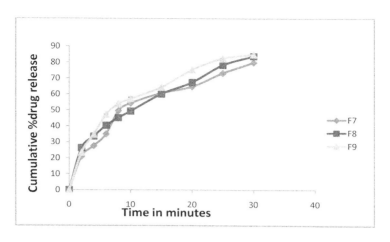

Figure 12. Graphical representation of Cumulative percent Tolterodine Tartrate released from ODTs containing varying concentrations of sodium starch glycolate.

Table 15. Formula of Tolterodine TartrateODTs prepared with combination of superdisintegrants.

Ingredients*	CP+SSG			CP + CCS			CCS + SSG		
	4%	6%	8%	4%	6%	8%	4%	6%	8%
Drug -polymer complex	12	12	12	12	12	12	12	12	12
Pearlitol SD 200	8.0	8.0	8.0	8.0	8.0	8.0	8.0	8.0	8.0
Avicel pH 101	52	50.4	48.8	52	50.4	48.8	52	50.4	48.8
Super disintegrants	3.2	4.8	6.4	3.2	4.8	6.4	3.2	4.8	6.4
Sodium saccharine (2%)	1.6	1.6	1.6	1.6	1.6	1.6	1.6	1.6	1.6
Orange flavor (2%)	1.6	1.6	1.6	1.6	1.6	1.6	1.6	1.6	1.6
Sodium stearylfumarate (0.25%)	0.8	0.8	0.8	0.8	0.8	0.8	0.8	0.8	0.8
Aerosil	0.8	0.8	0.8	0.8	0.8	0.8	0.8	0.8	0.8

Note: CP – Crosspovidone, CCS – Croscarmellose Sodium, SSG – Sodium Starch Glycolate

* All the amounts given in above table are in milligrams.

Table 16. Preformulation characteristics of Tolterodine TartrateODTs prepared with combinationofsuperdisintegrants

Formulation code	Bulk density (g/cc)	Tapped density (g/cc)	Hausner ratio	Compressibilty index (%)	Angle of repose
F10	0.380	0.452	1.18	15.29	27.65
F11	0.375	0.446	1.18	14.73	27
F12	0.369	0.439	1.17	14.98	29
F13	0.370	0.443	1.17	14.93	25
F14	0.380	0.446	1.17	14.83	26.25
F15	0.383	0.453	1.18	15.48	27
F16	0.370	0.442	1.19	15.45	28.54
F17	0.367	0.436	1.18	14.59	27.23
F18	0.379	0.456	1.20	15.48	24.87

Table 17. Tabletting characteristics of Tolterodine Tartrate ODTs prepared with combination of superdisintegrants

Formulation code	Hardness[a](kg/cm^2)	Friability[b] (%)	Weight[c] (mg)	Thickness[a] (mm)	Drug content[c](%)
F10	2.85±0.10	0.18	80.05±0.81	3.82±0.07	99.81±1.08
F11	3.0±0.06	0.36	79.87±0.79	3.83±0.008	98.20±0.31
F12	3.20±0.13	0.28	80.07±0.78	3.84±0.007	87.41±0.72
F13	2.41±0.07	0.24	79.94±0.97	3.82±0.01	102.00±0.21
F14	2.59±0.12	0.36	80.02±0.90	3.84±0.05	99.25±0.15
F15	3.17±0.22	0.28	79.90±0.92	3.84±0.008	100.84±1.41
F16	2.86±0.22	0.52	79.95±0.79	3.83±0.005	99.38±0.77
F17	3.27±0.07	0.29	79.90±0.79	3.79±0.01	99.65±1.42
F18	3.35±0.15	0.38	80.02±0.82	3.78±0.008	98.87±0.81

Table 18. Tabletting characteristics of Tolterodine Tartrate ODTs prepared with combination of superdisintegrants

Formulation	Disintegration time[a] (sec)	Wetting time[a] (sec)	Water absorption ratio[a] (%)	In vitro dispersion time[a] (sec)
F10	35.52±0.78	28.95±0.71	122.80±0.23	29.16±0.75
F11	29.71±0.44	42.58±0.49	115.42±0.56	25.83±0.75
F12	24.71±0.44	30.66±0.81	94.11±0.96	23.98±0.69
F13	20.16±0.75	28.48±0.44	125.59±0.6	21.43±0.22
F14	**15.02±0.40**	**19.20±0.22**	**142.69±0.98**	**16.19±0.55**
F15	17.46±0.40	23.45±0.77	136.82±0.17	18.27±0.81
F16	30.05±0.64	59.68±0.62	84.70±0.26	28.74±0.32
F17	47.63±0.52	47.55±1.40	69.81±0.24	32.07±0.54
F18	51.20±0.60	38.48±0.45	57.97±0.91	49.50±0.68

a: Mean±S.D., n=6 tablets, b: Mean±S.D., n=10 tablets, c: Mean±S.D., n=20 tablets.

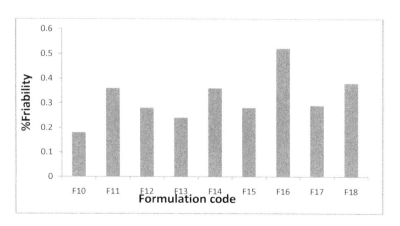

Figure 13. Graphical representation of friability of Tolterodine Tartrate ODTs prepared by varying concentrations of combination of superdisintegrants

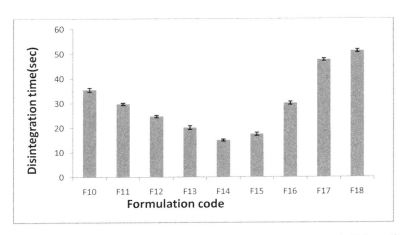

Figure 14. Graphical representation of disintegration times of Tolterodine Tartrate ODTs prepared by varying concentrations of combination of superdisintegrants

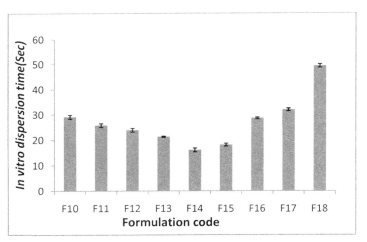

Figure 15. Graphical representation of in vitrodispersion time of Tolterodine TartrateODTs prepared by varying concentrations of combination of superdisintegrants

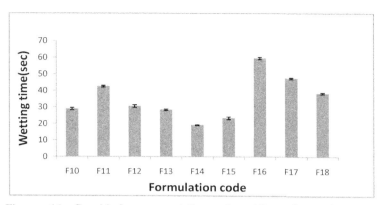

Figure 16 Graphical representation of wetting time of Tolterodine TartrateODTs prepared by varying concentrations of combination of superdisintegrants

Table 19. Cumulative percent Tolterodine Tartratereleased from ODTs prepared by varying concentrations of combination of superdisintegrants

Cumulative % drug release						
Time(min)	F10	F11	F12	F13	F14	F15
2	28.58±0.03	30.92±0.33	32.08±0.30	34.18±0.06	36.34±0.26	30.97±0.65
4	33.87±0.16	38.14±0.39	36.37±0.06	42.08±0.29	49.65±0.18	43.64±0.46
6	48.29±0.07	44.39±0.09	49.14±0.62	58.67±0.38	59.22±0.09	55.47±0.28
8	58.08±0.66	52.57±0.85	55.39±0.17	64.51±0.17	67.86±0.09	59.24±0.55
10	67.71±0.48	68.48±0.15	69.25±0.28	73.25±0.39	75.82±0.68	68.12±0.05
15	78.81±0.63	78.13±0.29	78.32±0.05	80.64±0.03	85.63±0.28	79.04±0.36
20	83.14±0.47	83.89±0.37	86.46±0.98	87.90±0.95	92.52±0.29	83.62±0.66
25	87.28±1.06	89.27±0.91	92.27±0.48	94.34±0.27	**99.65±0.45**	90.34±0.04
30	**94.80±0.32**	**95.50.±0.14**	**97.59±0.09**	**98.50±0.39**	**99.45±0.16**	**95.89±0.16**

Cumulative % drug release			
Time(min)	F16	F17	F18
2	26.28±0.06	28.14±0.47	25.28±0.41
4	29.58±0.09	32.02±0.46	29.48±0.26
6	36.21±0.25	39.72±0.09	38.57±0.49
8	48.54±0.68	45.14±0.87	57.37±0.25
10	56.04±0.29	57.72±0.03	64.14±0.08
15	66.72±0.30	62.97±1.06	68.17±0.98
20	79.36±0.03	74.26±0.56	77.62±0.84
25	80.38±0.37	80.15±0.34	84.91±0.76
30	85.79±0.50	89.50±0.18	90.49±0.69

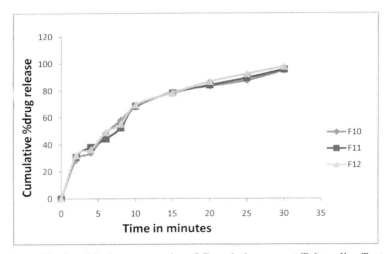

Figure 17. Graphical representation of Cumulative percent Tolterodine Tartrate released from ODTs containing varying concentrations of CP + SSG

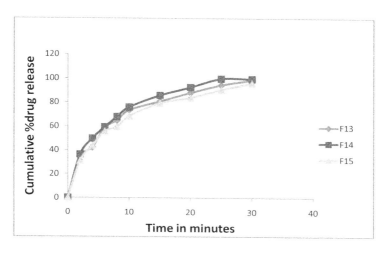

Figure 18. Graphical representation of Cumulative percent Tolterodine Tartrate released from ODTs containing varying concentrations of CP + CCS

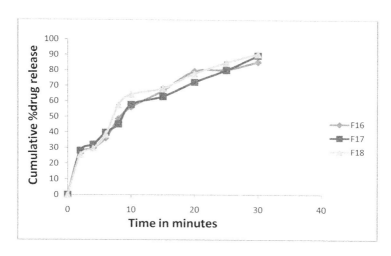

Figure 19. Graphical representation of Cumulative percent Tolterodine Tartrate released from ODTs containing varying concentrations of CCS + SSG

3.2.1. *In-vivo* Taste evaluation

Taste evaluation was performed on eight healthy human volunteers and the results were reported in the table 4.13. The bitterness of the drug was reduced or even masked after complexation with eudragit EPO in different ratios (1: 1, 1:2 and 1:3). In case of 1:1 ratio it was felt slightly metallic after 1 minute and it is apparent from the results that the increasing concentrations of the polymer have completely have completely masked the metallic taste of the drug. Since the drug is not in the native form and entrapped within the polymeric matrix, and there by reduction in the solubility of the drug in the saliva could have led to the masking of the b taste. Eventhough the Tolterodine Tartrate taste was masked with drug polymer complex (1:1, 1:2 and 1:3) ratioswe have selected 1:2 for further studies, since higher amounts of polymer may retard the dissolution performance of the final fast disintegrating tablets of Tolterodine Tartrate.

Table 20. Comparative taste evaluation

Degree of Bitterness					
Form of Tolterodine Tartrate	10 seconds	30 seconds	1 minute	2minutes	5minutes
DPC (1:1)	0	0	1	1	2
DPC (1:2)	0	0	0	1	0
DPC (1:3)	0	0	1	1	1
Optimized formulation	0	0	0	0	0

*Results are the mean of 3 observation

i.e. 0=tasteless, 1=slight bitter, 2=moderate bitter, 3=strong bitter.

3.2.2. *In vivo* Disintegration time

In Vivo disintegration was performed on eight healthy human volunteers. The subjects were informed of the purpose and protocol of the study. All volunteers were asked to rinse their mouth with distilled water prior to the test. Tablets were placed on the tongue and the time required for the complete disintegration of tablets was recorded (Table 3.14). Swallowing of saliva was prohibited during the test, and the mouth was rinsed after each measurement. This experiment was conducted in eight subjects and the mean±SD were calculated.

Table 21. *In Vivo* disintegration time evaluated in eight healthy human volunteers

Human volunteers	*In vivo* disintegration time(sec)
1	14
2	16
3	19
4	16
5	15
6	18
7	16
8	19

3.3. Fourier Transform Infrared Spectroscopy (FTIR) Studies

FTIR spectra of IR spectrum of pure Tolterodine Tartrate, croscarmellose sodium, crosspovidone, sodium starch glycolate and combination thereof were recorded on Perkin Elmer spectrophotometer. The scans were evaluated for presence of principle peaks of drug, shifting and masking of drug peaks due to presence of polymer. The FTIR spectra of pure Tolterodine Tartrate, crosspovidone, Sodium starch glycolate and combination thereof shown in following figures.

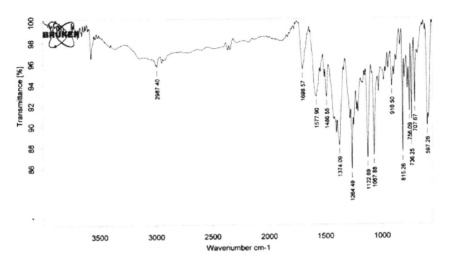

Figure 20. FTIR spectra of Tolterodine Tartrate

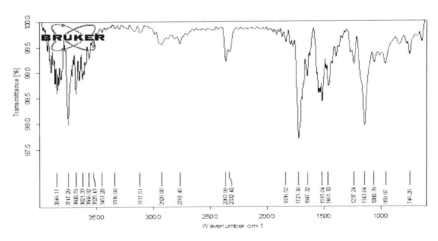

Figure 21. FTIR spectra of Eudragit polymer

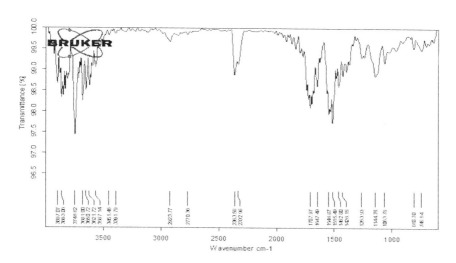

Figure 22. FTIR spectra of Tolterodine + Eudragit

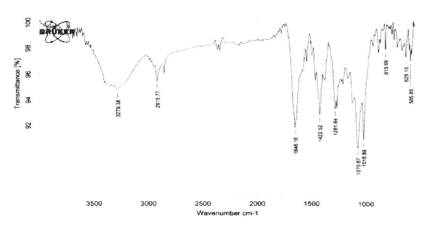

Figure 23 FTIR Spectra of Tolterodine + Crosspovidone

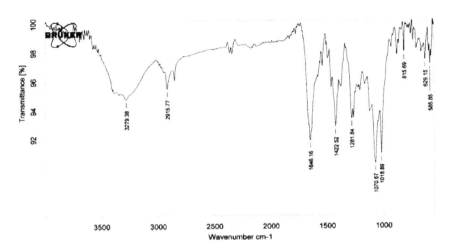

Figure 24. FTIR spectra of Tolterodine + croscarmellose sodium

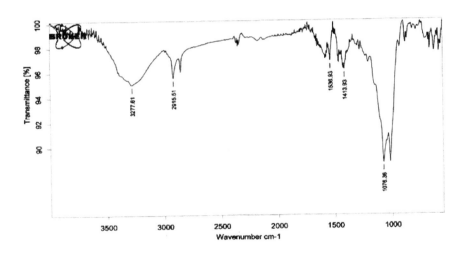

Figure 25. FTIR spectra of Tolterodine + Sodium starch glycolate

Figure 4.23: FTIR spectra of

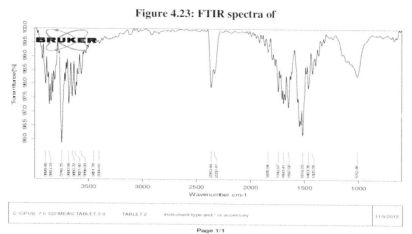

Figure 26. FTIR spectra of Tolterodine + tablet blend

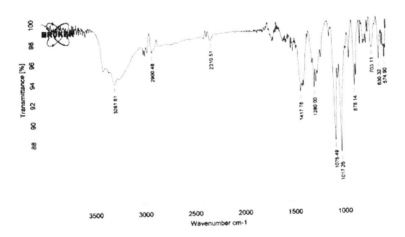

Figure 22. FTIR spectra of Tolterodine + pearlitol

IR Spectra	Peak of Functional groups [Wave length (cm-1)]				
	C-H Stretching (Alkane)	C=O Stretching (Phenols)	C-O Stretching (ester)	C=C Stretching (aromatic)	C-N Stretching (amide)
Tolterodine Tartrate	2987.40	1698.57	1264.49	3210.67	1122.69
Tolterodine + Eudragit EPO	2923	1647	1263	3298	1083
Tolterodine + CCS	2920	1689	1250	3278	1080
Tolterodine + CP	2915	1646	1281	3279	1070
Tolterodine + SSG	2915	1680	1210	3277	1076
Tolterodine + Blend	2931	1647	1210	3281	1012
Tolterodine + Perlitol	2900	1700	1280	3281	1075

The above peaks were considered as characteristics peaks of TolterodineTartrate. These peaks were not affected and prominently observed in IR spectra of drug and excipients. This indicates there is no interaction between drug and excipients.

4. DISCUSSION

The present investigation was under taken to formulate and evaluate oral disintegrating or disperse tablets in the saliva within a matter of seconds which overcome the swallowing problems and improves patient compliance.

Using various disintegrants like Crospovidone, Croscarmellose sodium, Sodium starch glycolate tablets were prepared along with other additives. Direct compression method was used for the preparation of tablets. A total number of 18 formulations were prepared and evaluated.

To achieve rapid disintegration time, most of the excipients selected must be water soluble by nature. Pearlitol SD 200 is a directly compressible grade of mannitol with good flow properties and gives a refreshing or cooling effect in the mouth due to its negative heat of solution. This excipient was used as a bulking agent to achieve the desired tablet weight.

Avicel 102 was included in the formulation mainly as a disintegrant at the concentrations used and to some extent as diluents. This grade of microcrystalline cellulose is powder in nature and thus displays excellent flow. To impart pleasant taste and mouth feel sodium saccharin and orangeflavour were included as sweetening and flavoring agents respectively. Sodium stearylfumarate was employed as a lubricant instead of magnesium stearate to overcome the metallic taste of the latter and also due to its water soluble nature.

Crospovidone polymers are densely crosslinkedhomopolymers of N – vinyl 2 – pyrrolidones. Their porous particle morphology helps to rapidly wick liquids into the tablet by capillary action to generate the rapid volume expansion and hydrostatic pressures that cause tablet disintegration. In addition to its unique particle size and morphology, crospovidoneis non ionic and its disintegration performance will neither be influenced by pH changes in the gastrointestinal tract nor will they complex with ionic drug actives. They can also be used as solubility enhancers resulting in a faster dissolution rate without forming gels.

Croscarmellose sodium is crosslinkedcarboxymethyl cellulose sodium which can be used at concentrations of upto 5% as a disintegrant. Its unique fibrous nature gives excellent water wicking capabilities and crosslinking makes it hydrophilic and highly absorbent material, resulting in its swelling properties. It rapidly swells upto 4 - 8 times its original volume on contact with water. Like crosspovidone, it is also used as a dissolution aid, hence the name Ac-Di-Sol (accelerates dissolution).

Sodium starch glycolate is a sodium salt of carboxymethyl ether of starch,usually employed at concentrations between 2 – 8% although an optimum concentration of 4% may sufficient in many cases. Disintegration occurs by rapid uptake of water followed by rapid and enormous swelling, which is its primary mechanism of action. It swells upto 300 times its original volume in water.

Pre-formulation studies:

The results obtained by evaluating the powder blends of drug and excipients are shown in table.Bulk density and tapped density were found in the range of 0.372-0.385g/cc and 0.436 – 0.465 g/cc respectively. The value ofhausner was in between 1.17 – 1.20 (< 1.25) indicating that all batches of powder blends were having good compressibility, Values of angle of repose (θ) was foundin the range of 25.54– 29 showing that blend of powder was free flowing and can be used for direct compression.

Weight variation and Thickness

In all formulations, tablet weight and thickness were within mean ±7.5% and mean ±5% respectively. The average weight in all the eighteen formulations was found to be 79.54±0.77 mg to 80.10±0.87mg. The thickness varies between 3.72 ± 0.02 to 3.84 ± 0.07mm.

Friability and Hardness

Friability values were less than 1% in all cases. Hardness of all the tablets was maintained at 2.46±0.40 to 3.5 ± 0.25 kg/cm^2 for all the formulations as mentioned before.

Assay

Assay was performed and percent drug content of all the tablets were found to be between 89.23± 1.22% and 102.00 ± 0.21% of TolterodineTartrate which was within the acceptable limits.

Wetting time

Wetting time was determined for all the formulations. The value lies between 19.20± 0.98to 59.68± 0.62sec. The variability in wetting time for different formulations may be due to the changes in the compaction which cannot be controlled during tablet preparation and the type of the disintegrant affected the wetting of the tablets. On comparing the superdisintegrantsthe formulations containingcrosspovidone + croscarmellose sodium and crossprovidone + sodium starch glycolatetake less wetting time than the other formulations containing single superdisintegrants.

Water absorption ratio

Water absorption ratio ranged from 37.30± 0.46 % to 142.69± 0.98 %. Crosspovidone and crosscarmellose sodium perform their disintegrating action by wicking through capillary action and fibrous structure, respectively with minimum gelling. The relative ability of the various disintegrants to wick water into the tablets was studied. After contact with water the tablets containing sodium starch glycolate swelled, the outer edge appeared gel like. Tablets containing crosscarmellose sodium quickly wicks water and were hydrated, but were soft as compared with tablets prepared with crosspovidone and sodium starch glycolate. The center of the tablets withcrosspovidon and sodium starch glycolateremained dry and hard.

Disintegration time

Disintegration time is considered to be important criteria in selecting the best ODT formulation. The *in vitro* disintegration time for all the 18 formulations varied from 15.02±0.40 to 52.66± 1.50 seconds. The rapid disintegration was seen in the formulations containing croscarmellosesodium and formulations containing combination of superdisintegrants (CP + CCS, CP + SSG). This is due to rapid uptake of the water from the medium, swelling and burst effect. It is also noticed that as the disintegrant concentration was increased from 4 to 8% the time taken for disintegration was reduced. The disintegration time of formulation (F14) containing 6% CCS+ 6% CP was found to be lower (15.02± 0.40) and was selected as the best ODT formulation among all the 18 formulations.

In vitro dispersion

In vitro dispersion is a special parameter in which the time taken by the tablet for complete dispersion is measured. The time for all the 18 formulations varied between 16.19± 0.55 and 59.83± 0.88 sec.

In vitro dissolution

The development of dissolution method for ODTs is almost similar to the approach taken for conventional tablets until they utilize the taste masking. The taste masking aspect greatly influences dissolution method development, specifications, and testing. Several factors like varied thickness and pH dependent solubility of drug particle coating influence dissolution profiles of ODTs containing taste masked actives. Since Tolterodine Tartrate is not bitter in taste, the bland taste of drug was masked by using sweeteners and flavors. It has been reported that USP type II apparatus with a paddle speed of 50 rpm is commonly used for ODTs formulations. Slower paddle speeds are utilized to obtain good profiles as these formulations disintegrate rapidly.

In vitro dissolution studies of the prepared ODTs was performed in mixture of solvent pH 6.8 phosphate buffer using USP dissolution apparatus type 2. The dissolution rate was found to increase linearly with increasing concentration of superdisintegrant. Formulations F1, F2 and F3which contained increasing concentrations of crosspovidon have recorded drug release 89.8±34.25%,90.57±0.44% and93.90±0.45% respectively within 30 min. Formulations F4, F5 and F6 which contained increasing concentrations of croscarmellose sodium have recorded drug release 93.88 ± 0.21%, 95.33± 1.27% and97.89 ± 0.28%

respectively, at the end of 30 min. Formulations F7, F8 and F9 which contained increasing concentrations of sodium starch glycolate have recorded drug release$79.89\pm0.17\%$, $83.85\pm0.52\%$ and $84.95\pm0.49\%$ respectively, at the end of 30 min.

Formulations F10, F11 and F12 which contained increasing concentrations of combination of CP+ SSG have recorded drug release$94.80\pm0.32\%$, $95.50\pm0.14\%$ and $97.59\pm0.09\%$ respectively, at the end of 30 min. Formulations F13, F14, and F15 which contained increasing concentrations of combination of CP + CCS have recorded drug release$98.50\pm0.39\%$,$99.65\pm0.45\%$,and95.89 ± 0.16 at the end of 25 to 30 min.

Formulations F16, F17 and F18 which contained increasing concentrations of combination of CCS + SSG have recorded drug release respectively, , $85.79 \pm 0.50\%$, $89.50 \pm 0.18\%$ and $90.49\pm 0.69\%$ at the end of 30 min.

Drug content:

Assay was performed and percent drug content of all the batches were found to be 104.19 ± 0.71, 99.40 ± 0.74 and 101.82 ± 0.16 of Tolterodine Tartrate which was within the acceptable limits.

5. CONCLUSION

Tolterodine Tartrate Oral Disintegrating Tablets were prepared by direct compression method using crosspovidone, croscarmellose sodium, sodium starch glycolate and combinations of, CP + SSG and CP+ CCS and CCS+SSG as superdisintegrants exhibited good preformulation and tabletting properties. Results demonstrated that 1:2 ratio of drug polymer complex completely masked the metallic taste, and formulated as orally disintegrating tablets with sufficient mechanical strength and desirable taste. F14 formulation containing 6% crosspovidon and croscarmellose sodium exhibited lowest disintegration time and rapid drug release compared to other superdisintegrants. Taste evaluation studies revealed that the metallic taste of Toltarodine Tartrate was completely masked by using eudragit EPO *in-vitro* and *in-vivo* disintegration time of F14 formulation was found to be almost similar. The above used superdisintegrants, formulation containing croscarmellose sodium(F6) and combination of CP + CCS (F14) showed better performance in terms of disintegration time and drug release when compared to other formulations.

- Order of the superdisintegrant activity is as follows

    (CP + CCS) > CCS > CP > (CP+ SSG) > (CCS + SSG) > SSG

- Oral Disintegrating Tablets were found to improve the versatility, convenience, patient compliance leading to an enhanced approach for the administration of drug to the pediatric and gediatrics

REFERENCES

Abdelbary, A., Elshafeey, A. H., and Zidan, G., Comparative effects of different cellulosic-based directly compressed orodispersable tablets on oral bioavailability of famotidine. *Carbohydrate polymers.*, 77, 799-806 (2009).

Adamo, F., Valentina, B., Gian, C.C., Celestino, R., Carlos ,A, F, M., Fast dispersible/slow releasing ibuprofen tablets. *Eur. J. Pharm. Biopharm.*, 69, 335–341 (2008).

Andreas, P., and Thomas, F., Pioglitazone: an antidiabetic drug with the potency to reduce cardiovascular mortality. *Expert Opin. Pharmacother.*, 7, 463-476 (2006).

Ashwini, R., Mangesh, R., and Rahul, R., Formulation Design and Optimization of Novel Taste Masked Mouth-Dissolving Tablets of Tramadol Having Adequate Mechanical Strength. *AAPS PharmSciTech.*, 10, 574-581 (2009).

Battu, S. K., Michael, A. R., Soumyajit, M., and Madhusudan, Y., Formulation and evaluation of rapidly disintegrating fenoverine tablets: Effect of superdisintegrants. *Drug Dev. Ind. Pharm.*, 33. 1225-1232 (2007).

Bhatu, P. B., and Atish, M., The technologies used for developing orally disintegrating tablets: A review. *Acta Pharm.*, 61, 117–139 (2011).

Chattopadhyay, R. R., and Bandyopadhyay, M., Effect of Azadirachta indica leaf extract on serum lipid profile changes in normal and streptozotocin induced diabetic rats. *Afr. J. Biomed. Research.*, 8, 101-104 (2005).

Chang, R.K., Guo, X., Burnside, B., Couch, R., Fast-dissolving tablets. *Pharm. Technol.*, 24, 52-58 (2000).

Debjit, B., Chiranjib, B., Krishnakanth., Pankaj., Margret, R., Fast Dissolving Tablets: An Overiew. *Journal. Chem. Pharm. Research.*, 1(1), 163 – 177 (2009).

Dobetti, L., Fast-Melting Tablets: Developments and Technologies. *Pharm. Technol. Drug Del. Suppl.*, 3, 44-50 (2001).

Francesco, C., Elisa, C., Paola, M., Susanna, B., Chiara, G., and Luisa, M., Diclofenac fast-dissolving film: suppression of bitterness by a taste-sensing system. *Drug Dev. Ind. Pharm.*, 37, 252–259 (2011).

Ganesan, K., Gani, S. B., and Arunachalam, G. M., Anti-diabetic Activity of *Helicteres isora* L. Bark Extracts on Streptozotocin-induced Diabetic Rats. *Int. J. Pharm Sci. Nano. Technol.*, 1, 379-382 (2009).

Goel, H., Arora, A., Tiwary, A. K., and Rana, V., Development and evaluation of mathematical model to predict disintegration time of fast disintegrating tablets using powder characteristics. *Pharm. Dev. Technol.*, 16, 57-64 (2011).

Guptha, A., Mishra, A. K., Guptha, V., Bansal, P., Singh, R., and Singh, A. K., Recent Trends of Fast Dissolving Tablet – An Overview of Formulation Technology. *Int. J. Pharm. Bio. Arch.*, 1 (1), 1 – 10 (2010).

James, K., Dissolution testing of orally disintegrating tablets. *Diss.Tech.*,10(2), 6-8 (2003).

Jianchen, X., Li, B., and Kang, Z., Taste masking microspheres for orally disintegrating tablets. *Int. J. Pharm.*, 359, 63-69 (2008).

Jinichi, F., Etsuo, Y., Yasuo, Y., and Katsuhide, T., Evaluation of rapidly disintegrating tablets containing glycine and carboxymethylcellulose. *Int. J. Pharm.*, 310, 101-109 (2006).

Kayitarea, E., Vervaet, C., Mehuys, E., Kayumba, P.C., Ntawukulilyayo, J., Karemac, C., Bortel, V., Remon, J. P., Taste-masked quinine pamoate tablets for treatment of children with uncomplicated Plasmodium falciparum malaria. *Int. J. Pharm.*, 392, 29–34 (2010).

Kuchekar, B. S., Arumugam, V., Formulation and evaluation of Metronidazole orodispersible tablets. *Indian J. Pharm. Edu.*, 35, 150-158 (2001).

Kuldeep, M., Kevin, G., Biswajit, B., Ravi, B., Bhavik, J., Narayana, R., An emerging trend in oral drug delivery technology: Rapid disintegrating tablets. *J. Pharm. Sci. Tech.*, 2 (10), 318 -329 (2010).

Kuno, Y., Kojima, M, Ando, S., Nakagami, H., Evaluation of rapidly disintegrating tablets manufactured by phase transition of sugar alcohols. *J Control Release.*, 105, 16-22 (2005).

Li, Q., Wei, W., Xiaofeng, C., Tao, Hu., Evaluation of Disintegrating Time of Rapidly Disintegrating Tablets by a Paddle Method. *Pharm. Dev. Technol.*, 11, 295–301 (2006).

Manoj, W., Kothawade, P., Kishore, S., Nayana, V., and Vandana, D., Techniques used in orally disintegrating drug delivery system. *Int. J. Drug. Delivery*: 2, 98 – 107 (2010).

Mizumoto, T., Tamura, T., Kawai, H., Kajiyama, A., and Itai, S., Formulation Design of Taste-Masked Particles, Including Famotidine, for an Oral Fast-Disintegrating Dosage Form. *Chem. Pharm. Bull.*, 56, 530-535 (2008).

Morella, A. M., Pitman, I. H., Heinicke, G. W., Taste masked liquid suspensions. *US Patent.*, 6,197,348 (2001).

Morita, Y., Tsuhima, Y., Yasui, M., Termoz, R., Ajioka, J., and Takayam, K., Evaluation of the disintegration time of rapidly disintegrating tablets via a novel method utilizing CCD camera. *Chem. Pharm. Bull.*, 50 (9), 1181-1186 (2002).

Nanda, A., Kandarapu, R., Garg. S., An update on taste masking technologies for oral pharmaceuticals. *Indian J. Pharm. Sci.*, 64, 10-17 (2002).

Nishant, V., and Vikas, R., Preparation and optimization of mouth/orally dissolving tablets using a combination of glycine, carboxymethyl cellulose and sodium alginate: A Comparison with Superdisintegrants. *Pharm. Dev. Technol.*, 13, 233-243 (2008).

Nitin, S., Sanjula, B., Alka, A., Javed, Al., Fast-dissolving intra-oral drug delivery systems. *Expert Opin. Ther. Patents.*, **18**(7), 769-781(2008).

Okuda, Y., Irisawa, Y., Okimoto, K., Osawa, T., and Yamashita, S., A new formulation for orally disintegrating tablets using a suspension spray-coating method. *Int. J. Pharm.*, 382 : 80–87 (2009).

Piera, D. M., Sante, M., Pascal, W., Evaluation of Different Fast Melting Disintegrants by Means of a Central Composite. *Design. Drug. Dev. Ind. Pharm.*, 31,109–121(2005).

Puttewar, T., Kshirsagar, M., Chandewar, A. V., Chikhale, R., Formulation and evaluation of orodispersible tablet of taste masked doxylamine succinate using ion exchange resin. *J. K.Saud Univ.*, 22, 229–240 (2010).

Rangasamy, M., Oral disintegrating tablets: A future compaction. *Int. J. Pharm. Res. Dev.*, 1(10), 1-10 (2009).

Rajan, K., and Sanjay, G., Current Status of Drug Delivery Technologies and Future Directions. *Pharm. Tech.*, 25 (2), 1–14 (2001).

Rakesh, P., Mona, P., Prabodh, C., Sharma., Dhirender, K., and Sanju, N., Orally Disintegrating Tablets – Friendly to Pediatrics and Geriatrics. *Arch. Pharm. Res.*, 2 (2), 35 – 48 (2010).

Rikka, L., Eero, S., Mikko, B., Joakim, R., Vesa, P. L., Kristiina, J., and Jarkko, K., Perphenazine solid dispersions for orally fast-disintegrating tablets: physical stability and formulation. *Drug Dev. Ind. Pharm.*, 36, 601-613 (2010).

Rosie, M. L., Susan, B., and Kieran, C., Orally Disintegrating Tablets: The Effect of Recent FDA Guidance on ODT Technologies and Applications. *Pharm. Technol.*, 1-6 (2009).

Seong, J. H., and Kinam, P., Development of sustained release fast-disintegrating tablets using various polymer-coated ion-exchange resin complexes. *Int. J. Pharm.*, 353, 195-204 (2008).

Shagufta, K., Prashant, K., Premchand, N., and Pramod, Y., Taste Masking of Ondansetron Hydrochloride by Polymer Carrier System and Formulation of Rapid-Disintegrating Tablets. *AAPS Pharm Sci Tech.*, 8, 1-7 (2007).

Shery, J., Arun, S., and Anroop, N., Preparation and evaluation of fast disintegrating effervescent tablets of glibenclamide. *Drug Dev. Ind. Pharm.*, 35, 321-328 (2009).

Shirwaikar, A. A., Fast Disintegrating Tablets of Atenolol by Dry Granulation Method. *Ind. J. Pharm. Sci.*, 66(4), 422-426 (2004).

Shoukri, R., Ahmed, S., and Shamma, N., In-vitro and in-vivo evaluation of nimesulide lyophilized orally disintegrating tablets. *Eur. J. Pharm. Sci.*, 73, 162–171 (2009).

Shukla, D., Subhashis, C., Sanjiv., Brahmeshwar, M., Mouth Dissolving Tablets II: An Overview of Evaluation Techniques. *Sci Pharm.*, 77, 327 – 341 (2009).

Sohi, H., Sultana, Y., Khar, R. K., Taste masking technologies in oral pharmaceuticals: Recent developments and approaches. *Drug Dev. Ind. Pharm.*, 30, 429-448 (2004).

Suhas, M., Kakade., Vinodh, S., Mannur, Ketan., Ramani, B., Ayaz, A., Dhada., Chirag., Naval, V., Avinash, B., Formulation and Evaluation of Mouth dissolving tablets of Losartan potassium by direct compression techniques. *Int. J. Res. Pharm. Sci.*, 1(3), 290-295 (2010).

Suresh, B., Rajender, M., Ramesh, G., Madhusudan Rao, Y., Orodispersible tablets: An overview. *Asian J Pharm.*, 2(1), 2-11 (2008).

Tansel, C., Aysegul, D., Seluck, C., and Nursabah, B., Formulation and evaluation of diclofenac potassium fast-disintegrating tablets and their clinical application in migraine patients. *Drug Dev. Ind. Pharm.*, 37, 260-267 (2011).

Tejvir, K., Bhawandeep, G., Sandeep., and Guptha, G.D., Mouth Dissolving Tablets: A Novel Approach to Drug Delivery. *Int. J. Curr. Pharm. Res.*, 3 (1), 1-7 (2011).

Uday, S., Rangole., Kawtikwar, P. S., and Sakarkar, D. M., Formulation and In - vitro Evaluation of Rapidly Disintegrating Tablets using Hydrochlorothiazide as a model drug. *Research J. Pharm and Tech.*, 349 – 352 (2008).

William, R.P., Tapash, K., Orally disintegrating tablets. *Pharma. Tech.* (Product, Technologies and Development issues in Oct 2005).

Wipada, S., Praneet, O., Prasert, A., Tanasait, N., Kaewnapa, W., and Suwannee, P., Preparation and evaluation of taste-masked dextromethorphan oral disintegrating tablet. *Pharm. Dev. Technol.*, 1-6 (2011).

Xiao, N., Jin, S., Xiaopeng, H., Wu, Y., Zhongtian, Y., Jihong, H., and Zhonggui, H., Strategies to improve dissolution and oral absorption of glimepiride tablets: solid dispersion versus micronization techniques. *Drug Dev. Ind. Pharm.*, 1–10 (2010).

Xua, J., Bovet, L., Zhao, K., Taste masking microspheres for orally disintegrating tablets. *Int. J. Pharm.*, 359, 63–69 (2008).

Yourong, F., Shicheng, Y., Seong, J. H., Susumu, K., and Kinam, P., Orally Fast Disintegrating Tablets: Developments, Technologies, Taste-Masking and Clinical Studies. *Crit Rev Ther Drug Carrier Sys.*, 21, 433–475 (2004).

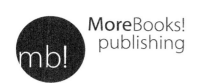
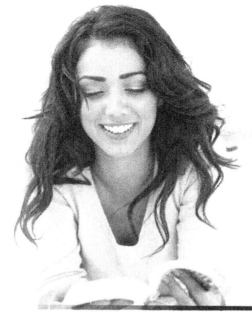

i want morebooks!

Buy your books fast and straightforward online - at one of world's fastest growing online book stores! Environmentally sound due to Print-on-Demand technologies.

Buy your books online at
www.get-morebooks.com

Kaufen Sie Ihre Bücher schnell und unkompliziert online – auf einer der am schnellsten wachsenden Buchhandelsplattformen weltweit! Dank Print-On-Demand umwelt- und ressourcenschonend produziert.

Bücher schneller online kaufen
www.morebooks.de

VDM Verlagsservicegesellschaft mbH
Heinrich-Böcking-Str. 6-8
D - 66121 Saarbrücken

Telefon: +49 681 3720 174
Telefax: +49 681 3720 1749

info@vdm-vsg.de
www.vdm-vsg.de

Printed in Great Britain
by Amazon